OPPOSING VIEWPOINTS®

HEALTH

Other Books of Related Interest

OPPOSING VIEWPOINTS®

HEALTH

Auriana Ojeda, *Book Editor*

Daniel Leone, *President*
Bonnie Szumski, *Publisher*
Scott Barbour, *Managing Editor*
Helen Cothran, *Senior Editor*

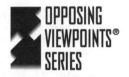

OPPOSING
VIEWPOINTS®
SERIES

GREENHAVEN
PRESS®

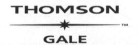

THOMSON
———————
GALE

San Diego • Detroit • New York • San Francisco • Cleveland
New Haven, Conn. • Waterville, Maine • London • Munich

JAN 2 7 2004

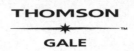

LIBRARY OF CONGRESS CATALOGING-IN-PUBLICATION DATA

Health / Auriana Ojeda, book editor.
    p. cm. — (Opposing viewpoints series)
Includes bibliographical references and index.
ISBN 0-7377-1684-3 (lib. : alk. paper) — ISBN 0-7377-1683-5 (pbk. : alk. paper)
    1. Health—Miscellanea. I. Ojeda, Auriana, 1977– . II. Series.
RA776.H434 2004
613—dc21   2003054045

Printed in the United States of America

"Congress shall make
no law...abridging the
freedom of speech, or of
the press."

First Amendment to the U.S. Constitution

The basic foundation of our democracy is the First
Amendment guarantee of freedom of expression.
The Opposing Viewpoints Series is dedicated to the
concept of this basic freedom and the idea that it is
more important to practice it than to enshrine it.

Contents

Why Consider
Opposing Viewpoints?

*"The only way in which a human being can make some
approach to knowing the whole of a subject is by hearing
what can be said about it by persons of every variety of
opinion and studying all modes in which it can be looked
at by every character of mind. No wise man ever
acquired his wisdom in any mode but this."*

John Stuart Mill

In our media-intensive culture it is not difficult to find differing opinions. Thousands of newspapers and magazines
and dozens of radio and television talk shows resound with
differing points of view. The difficulty lies in deciding which
opinion to agree with and which "experts" seem the most
credible. The more inundated we become with differing
opinions and claims, the more essential it is to hone critical
reading and thinking skills to evaluate these ideas. Opposing
Viewpoints books address this problem directly by present-
ing stimulating debates that can be used to enhance and
teach these skills. The varied opinions contained in each
book examine many different aspects of a single issue. While
examining these conveniently edited opposing views, readers
can develop critical thinking skills such as the ability to
compare and contrast authors' credibility, facts, argumenta-
tion styles, use of persuasive techniques, and other stylistic
tools. In short, the Opposing Viewpoints Series is an ideal
way to attain the higher-level thinking and reading skills so
essential in a culture of diverse and contradictory opinions.

   In addition to providing a tool for critical thinking, Opposing Viewpoints books challenge readers to question their
own strongly held opinions and assumptions. Most people
form their opinions on the basis of upbringing, peer pressure, and personal, cultural, or professional bias. By reading
carefully balanced opposing views, readers must directly
confront new ideas as well as the opinions of those with
whom they disagree. This is not to simplistically argue that

everyone who reads opposing views will—or should—change his or her opinion. Instead, the series enhances readers' understanding of their own views by encouraging confrontation with opposing ideas. Careful examination of others' views can lead to the readers' understanding of the logical inconsistencies in their own opinions, perspective on why they hold an opinion, and the consideration of the possibility that their opinion requires further evaluation.

Evaluating Other Opinions

To ensure that this type of examination occurs, Opposing Viewpoints books present all types of opinions. Prominent spokespeople on different sides of each issue as well as well-known professionals from many disciplines challenge the reader. An additional goal of the series is to provide a forum for other, less known, or even unpopular viewpoints. The opinion of an ordinary person who has had to make the decision to cut off life support from a terminally ill relative, for example, may be just as valuable and provide just as much insight as a medical ethicist's professional opinion. The editors have two additional purposes in including these less known views. One, the editors encourage readers to respect others' opinions—even when not enhanced by professional credibility. It is only by reading or listening to and objectively evaluating others' ideas that one can determine whether they are worthy of consideration. Two, the inclusion of such viewpoints encourages the important critical thinking skill of objectively evaluating an author's credentials and bias. This evaluation will illuminate an author's reasons for taking a particular stance on an issue and will aid in readers' evaluation of the author's ideas.

It is our hope that these books will give readers a deeper understanding of the issues debated and an appreciation of the complexity of even seemingly simple issues when good and honest people disagree. This awareness is particularly important in a democratic society such as ours in which people enter into public debate to determine the common good. Those with whom one disagrees should not be regarded as enemies but rather as people whose views deserve careful examination and may shed light on one's own.

Thomas Jefferson once said that "difference of opinion leads to inquiry, and inquiry to truth." Jefferson, a broadly educated man, argued that "if a nation expects to be ignorant and free . . . it expects what never was and never will be." As individuals and as a nation, it is imperative that we consider the opinions of others and examine them with skill and discernment. The Opposing Viewpoints Series is intended to help readers achieve this goal.

David L. Bender and Bruno Leone,
Founders

Greenhaven Press anthologies primarily consist of previously published material taken from a variety of sources, including periodicals, books, scholarly journals, newspapers, government documents, and position papers from private and public organizations. These original sources are often edited for length and to ensure their accessibility for a young adult audience. The anthology editors also change the original titles of these works in order to clearly present the main thesis of each viewpoint and to explicitly indicate the opinion presented in the viewpoint. These alterations are made in consideration of both the reading and comprehension levels of a young adult audience. Every effort is made to ensure that Greenhaven Press accurately reflects the original intent of the authors included in this anthology.

Introduction

"People are getting messages [about nutrition] from the left and right, often about just the latest findings from a new study, and that's not usually sufficiently reliable . . . , and that can make what is even at best a complicated story really very confusing."
    —*Walter Willett*, MSNBC News, *April 21, 2003.*

Americans are among the most unhealthy people in the world. According to the Centers for Disease Control and Prevention, almost two-thirds of Americans—approximately 97.1 million adults and 6.7 million children and teens—are overweight. The number of overweight Americans has more than tripled in the last twenty years. In addition to high rates of obesity, Americans suffer higher rates of heart disease and cancer than people living in any other country in the world. Cardiovascular disease is the number one cause of death in America, and at least 58 million Americans experience some form of heart disease. Cancer is the second highest cause of death in the United States, resulting in more than five hundred thousand deaths per year.

Despite the fact that rates of obesity, cardiovascular disease, and cancer are rising, the sorry state of American health is not new. Health experts have admonished people to eat healthy foods and to exercise since the 1950s, but the incidence of "lifestyle diseases"—noncommunicable diseases related to unhealthy lifestyles and unbalanced diets—continues to increase. Since many health problems are related to a poor diet, government health departments have issued numerous guidelines over the last fifty years to help the public navigate the bewildering abundance of food choices. However as new research about the causes of lifestyle diseases surfaces, the guidelines quickly become outdated. Thus, many people remain confused about which foods, and in what quantity, constitute a healthy diet.

In 1956 the U.S. Department of Agriculture (USDA) published a leaflet called *Food for Fitness—a Daily Food Guide*, in which it outlined the Four Basic Food Groups: 1) Meats, poultry, fish, beans and peas, eggs, and nuts; 2) dairy foods, including milk, cheese, and butter; 3) grains; 4) fruits and vegetables. These guidelines recommended that Americans prepare their meals from the Four Food Groups, relying heavily on the meat and dairy groups. The primary goal of the Four Food Groups was to ensure that Americans consumed sufficient vitamins, minerals, and other nutrients. Food producers enthusiastically endorsed the Four Food Groups because every one of their products had a place in the guidelines. Thus, they felt justified in promoting all foods as healthy, including foods that were high in fat and calories.

Unfortunately, many people began to complain that the Four Food Groups was primarily a campaign to promote the meat and dairy industries. As stated by nutritionist Neal D. Barnard, "Dairy products got their own group, and it was prominently featured. If you look at the fine print on the posters that are in schools, it indicates that the Dairy Council has put these out. They print the posters, and they still promote the old Four Food Groups because it increases sales of their products. It's the same with the meat producers." Despite questions about its reliability, the Four Food Groups guide remained the principal source for nutritional information until the 1970s.

By the 1970s a growing body of research began to associate overconsumption of certain food components—saturated fat, cholesterol, and sodium—with the risk of chronic diseases, such as heart disease and stroke. According to Harvey Levenstein, author of *Paradox of Plenty: The Social History of Eating in Modern America*, the government was slow to acknowledge the association between foods high in saturated fat and cholesterol—meat and dairy—and health problems because their research efforts were largely responsive to beef and dairy interests. However, nongovernmental health organizations, such as the American Heart Association and the American Cancer Society, pioneered aggressive research into the relationship between diet and health. As stated by Levenstein, "Not only did they subsidize research into the deleterious effects of various foods on their particular ailments, they also took the lead in disseminating any adverse results. They began spending millions to warn the public of the supposedly terrible consequences of eating foods containing too much sodium, sugar, and animal fats, as well as the perils of being overweight."

Thus began a new era in health education known as the Negative Nutrition or Selective Nutrition period. Instead of placing emphasis on eating enough nutrients, Negative Nutrition warned against eating certain kinds of foods. Dairy was a major target, because the cholesterol in milkfat and butterfat was believed to contribute to heart disease and other deadly illnesses. Sugar was also targeted as an addictive drug that was responsible for cancer, heart disease, diabetes, skin ailments, hyperactivity, and schizophrenia, among other mental and physical ailments. A few years later, meat products came under suspicion because they contained saturated fat, another contributor to heart disease. In 1977 the Senate published the *Dietary Goals for the United States*, which included new nutrition objectives, and within four years, Negative Nutrition became the core of national nutrition policy. In 1980, based on the Senate's *Dietary Goals*, the USDA published the *Dietary Guidelines for Americans*, a comprehensive nutritional reference guide that is updated every five years.

Food producers responded to the USDA's *Dietary Guidelines* by introducing hundreds of "low-fat," "low-calorie," "fat-free," "cholesterol-free," and "sodium-free" versions of their foods. To further confuse matters the Ronald Reagan administration lifted previous restrictions on advertising health claims, and advertisements for "heart-healthy" and "healthwise" products became the public's primary source for nutritional information. Unfortunately many food producers pandered to the demand for low-fat and low-cholesterol foods using false advertising. In response to the onslaught of unsubstantiated health claims on food labels, the government passed the Nutrition Labeling and Education Act (NLEA) in 1990. The act ensured that consumers had access to accurate nutritional information, including a list of the product's ingredients as well as the calorie, fat, sodium, cholesterol, and sugar content.

Soon after passing the NLEA, the USDA published an updated version of the Four Basic Food Groups guide, known as the *Food Guide Pyramid*, in 1992. The *Food Guide Pyramid*, which follows the *Dietary Guidelines for Americans*, pictures fruits, vegetables, and grains at its broad base, recommending six to eleven servings of grains and three to five servings of fruits and vegetables per day. The guide locates meat and dairy products on the next (smaller) section of the pyramid, recommending daily consumption of two to three servings from the meat and dairy groups. Last, the guidelines place oils, sweets, and fats at the narrowest tip of the pyramid, indicating that these foods should be used sparingly. As stated in the *Food Guide Pyramid Booklet*, "By following the *Dietary Guidelines*, you can enjoy better health and reduce your chances of getting certain diseases."

Many people disagree with the *Food Guide Pyramid* and argue that the guidelines still recommend excessive amounts of meat and dairy products. In 1992 the Physicians Committee for Responsible Medicine (PCRM), a health and nutrition advocacy group, unveiled its recommended New Four Food Groups guide. The New Four Food Groups recommends a diet based primarily on grains, vegetables, fruits, and legumes (or anything in a pod, such as beans, lentils, or peas). Many vegetarian organizations advocate the New Four Food Groups and contend that the foods suggested by these guidelines provide all the necessary nutrients for good health, contain no cholesterol, and are very low in fat. Supporters also argue that the low-fat content of these foods makes them especially valuable to ensure long-term weight management. As reported by PCRM, "The major killers of Americans—heart disease, cancer, and stroke—have a dramatically lower incidence among people consuming primarily plant-based diets. Weight problems—a contributor to a host of health problems—can also be brought under control by following the New Four Food Group recommendations."

The twentieth century saw remarkable discoveries in the field of health and nutrition, but the array of information available to guide consumers is bewildering. The conflicting information offered in the *Food Guide Pyramid* and the New Four Food Groups can be frustrating and discouraging for people trying to follow healthy lifestyles and avoid disease. Rather than struggling to adhere to a rigid set of regulations, many dietitians now maintain that a healthy diet incorporates the basic principles of variety, balance, and moderation. Thus, no food is taboo, so long as it is only eaten once in a while. As stated by the American Dietetic Association, "Rather than being taught to avoid certain foods, [people] should be taught ways to incorporate all foods into a healthy diet that is based on the principles of variety, balance, and moderation."

In *Health: Opposing Viewpoints*, authors examine the importance of a healthy diet and other issues related to health in the following chapters: What Factors Pose the Greatest Health Risks and Benefits? Are Exercise and Weight Loss Treatments Beneficial? Are Alternative Therapies Beneficial? How Can Government Policies Promote Good Health? Throughout these chapters, authors debate the issues that affect the health of all Americans.

CHAPTER 1

What Factors Pose the Greatest Health Risks and Benefits?

Chapter Preface

Health experts agree that drinking plenty of water is one of the most important factors in maintaining good health. Most dietary guidelines recommend drinking eight eight-ounce glasses of water per day. However, some researchers suggest that these recommendations may be inaccurate; instead of drinking eight glasses of plain water every day, many experts now contend that consuming about sixty-four ounces of any fluid daily meets the body's needs. The required fluid can be found in beverages other than water and in food, they argue. Regardless of how water is consumed, health researchers agree that plenty of fluid is vital to all sorts of bodily functions.

Water makes up about 50 to 80 percent of a person's body weight and contributes to proper blood flow, lubricates the joints and eyes, helps with swallowing, aids in waste disposal, and helps regulate body temperature through sweating. In addition, water maintains kidney health by helping flush toxins and body waste through them and reduces the risk of kidney or bladder stones. Research suggests that drinking plenty of water can reduce the risk of breast cancer and cancers of the colon and urinary tract. Moreover, some experts allege that drinking a lot of water can prevent obesity by creating a feeling of fullness and reducing the amount of food consumed in a meal. Since many people mistake feeling thirsty for feeling hungry, drinking water can reduce the amount of food eaten throughout the day.

The body continuously loses water through waste disposal, through the skin in the form of sweat, and from the lungs when people exhale. The lost water must be replaced or the body becomes dehydrated. Early signs of dehydration include headache, fatigue, loss of appetite, mental fogginess, flushed skin, light-headedness, and dry mouth and eyes. Nutritionists estimate that half of the American population is moderately dehydrated and attribute many common ailments, such as lethargy and muscle aches, to inadequate hydration. According to experts, most people consume liquids only when they are thirsty, but by the time most people are thirsty, they are already somewhat dehydrated. If dehydration becomes more advanced, people can experience difficulty swallowing, clumsiness, shriveled skin, sunken eyes, dim vision, painful urination, muscle spasms, and delirium.

Traditionally, health experts have suggested that people drink eight glasses of plain water every day to keep their bodies hydrated. However, researchers are now finding that beverages such as soda, coffee, tea, milk, and juice also satisfy the body's need for fluids. Noncaffeinated beverages contribute nearly as much fluid to the body as plain water; a glass of milk, for example, is about 90 percent water. Surprisingly some experts now contend that caffeinated beverages can be beneficial as well. Caffeine is a diuretic, which means that it draws water from the body to produce more urine. Therefore, according to traditional thinking, caffeinated beverages, such as coffee, tea, and soda sap the body of more fluid than they provide. Recently, however, experts learned that the amount of fluid lost as a result of consuming a diuretic beverage has been exaggerated. According to the *Tufts University Health & Nutrition Letter*, "You lose a significant amount of everything you drink, which is why you have to replenish the body with fluids every day. But you don't lose all the water in a cup of coffee, let alone the water in some other beverage you may have consumed before you drank the coffee." Thus, although caffeinated beverages provide less water than noncaffeinated beverages, they do not put the body at risk of dehydration.

Experts also maintain that food, especially fruits and vegetables, provides the body with a surprising amount of water. Researchers at Purdue University contend that iceberg lettuce, cucumbers, and celery, for example, are each about 95 percent water. Also, an orange is 87 percent water, and a banana is about 74 percent. Even a sirloin steak is about 59 percent water, and a slice of white bread is 37 percent water. Thus, according to these researchers, the water in food satisfies a large portion of the body's water needs.

To be sure, experts do not recommend relying solely on food to meet the body's fluid requirements. Nutritionists still suggest that people strive to consume eight glasses of liquid every day, but they also contend that eating a healthy diet full of fruits and vegetables will help satisfy the body's needs. As stated by Ruth Kava, the director of nutrition for the American College of Science and Health, "For many Americans—particularly those whose diets are high in fruits and vegetables—drinking a half-gallon of water [every day] is superfluous." Authors in the following chapter debate other factors that pose health risks and benefits.

*"More Americans are killed by cigarettes
than alcohol, car accidents, suicide, AIDS,
homicide, and illegal drugs."*

Smoking Is Dangerous to Human Health

American Cancer Society

In the following viewpoint the American Cancer Society
(ACS) asserts that smoking is the leading preventable cause
of death in the United States. According to the ACS, smoking contributes to lung cancer, heart disease, bronchitis, and
emphysema, among other ailments. The ACS contends that
quitting smoking greatly reduces a person's risk of contract-
ing cancer or other smoking-related diseases. The ACS is a
nationwide, community-based voluntary health organization dedicated to eliminating cancer as a major health problem by preventing cancer, saving lives, and diminishing suffering from cancer, through research, education, advocacy,
and service.

As you read, consider the following questions:
1. What kinds of cancers, besides lung cancer, does
   cigarette smoking cause, according to the ACS?
2. What three substances listed by the ACS are intended to
   enhance the smoking experience?
3. How does the author define addiction?

American Cancer Society, "Cigarette Smoking," www.cancer.org, October 18,
1999. Copyright © 1999 by the American Cancer Society. Reproduced by
permission.

The 1982 Surgeon General's Report stated "Cigarette smoking is the major single cause of cancer mortality in the United States." This statement is as true today as it was in 1982. Tobacco causes many types of cancer, and when cancer statistics are combined with all smoking-related diseases, cigarette use kills half of all continuing smokers.

More Americans are killed by cigarettes than alcohol, car accidents, suicide, AIDS, homicide, and illegal drugs.

Because cigarette smoking and tobacco use is an acquired behavior, one that the individual chooses to do, smoking is the most preventable cause of premature death in our society. In 2002, a staggering 430,700 deaths [were] expected in the U.S. from tobacco use. Yet, 46.5 million adults were current smokers in 2000.

Review of Cancers and Serious Illnesses Caused by Tobacco

Cigarette smoking is a major cause of cancers of the lung, larynx, oral cavity, pharynx and esophagus and is a contributing cause in the development of cancers of the bladder, pancreas, uterine cervix, kidney, stomach, and some leukemias.

About 87% of lung cancer deaths are caused by smoking. Lung cancer is one of the most difficult cancers to treat. It is very difficult to detect when it is in the earliest, most treatable stage. Fortunately, lung cancer is largely a preventable disease. Groups that advocate nonsmoking as part of their religion, such as Mormons and Seventh-day Adventists, have much lower rates of lung cancer and other smoking-related cancers.

Smoking is a major cause of heart disease, bronchitis, emphysema, and stroke and contributes to the severity of colds and pneumonia. Tobacco has a damaging effect on women's health and is associated with increased risk of miscarriage, preterm delivery, stillbirth, and infant death, and is a cause of low birth weight in infants. Furthermore, the secondhand smoke from cigarettes has a harmful health effect on those around the smoke.

Ingredients in Tobacco

Cigarettes, cigars, and smokeless and pipe tobacco consist of dried tobacco leaves, as well as ingredients added for flavor and other properties. More than 4,000 individual compounds have been identified in tobacco and tobacco smoke. Among these are about 43 compounds that are carcinogens.

There are hundreds of substances that are added by manufacturers to cigarettes to enhance the flavor or to make the smoking experience more pleasant. Some of the more common include ammonia, tar and carbon monoxide.

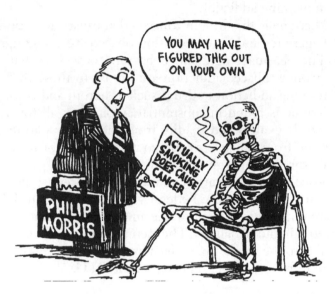

Wasserman. © 1999 by *Boston Globe*. Reprinted by permission of the Los Angeles Times Syndicate.

The Centers for Disease Control and Prevention recently developed a test to quantify flavor-related compounds in cigarette tobacco. Over sixty brands of cigarettes were tested, and 68% of the cigarettes contained at least one of 12 compounds, some of which are thought to be cancer-causing substances in animals. Exactly what effect these substances have on the cigarette consumer's health is unknown, but there is also no evidence that lowering the tar content of a cigarette improves the health risk. Manufacturers do not provide the public information about the precise amount of additives used in cigarettes, so it is difficult to accurately gauge that public health risk.

Nicotine Addiction

Addiction is characterized by the repeated, compulsive seeking or use of a substance despite harmful consequences. Addiction is often accompanied by adverse physical and psychological dependence on the substance. Nicotine is the addictive drug in tobacco. Regular use of tobacco products leads to addiction in a high proportion of users.

In 1988, the US Surgeon General concluded the following on nicotine addiction:

- Nicotine is the drug in tobacco that causes addiction.
- Cigarettes and other forms of tobacco are addicting.
- The pharmacologic and behavioral processes that determine tobacco addiction are similar to those that determine addiction to drugs such as heroin and cocaine.

Nicotine is found in substantial amounts in all forms of tobacco. It is absorbed readily from tobacco smoke in the lungs and from smokeless tobacco in the mouth or nose and rapidly spreads throughout the body.

Tobacco companies are required by law to report nicotine levels in cigarettes to the Federal Trade Commission (FTC) but are not required to show the amount of nicotine on the cigarette brand labeling. The actual amount of nicotine available to the smoker in a given brand of cigarettes may be different from the level reported to the FTC.

Health Benefits of Quitting

In September 1990, the US Surgeon General outlined the benefits of smoking cessation:

- People who quit, regardless of age, live longer than people who continue to smoke.
- Smokers who quit before age 50 have half the risk of dying in the next 15 years compared with those who continue to smoke. Those who quit by age 35 avoid 90% of the risk attributable to tobacco.
- Quitting smoking substantially decreases the risk of cancer of the lung, larynx, pharynx, esophagus, mouth, pancreas, bladder, and cervix.
- Benefits of cessation include risk reduction for other major diseases including coronary heart disease, lung diseases, and cardiovascular disease.

The risk of having lung cancer and other smoking-related cancers is related to total lifetime exposure to cigarette smoke, as measured by the number of cigarettes smoked each day, the age at which smoking began, and the number of years a person has smoked.

The risk increases steadily with the number of cigarettes smoked per day. In those who smoke 40 or more cigarettes a day (2 or more packs), the risk of lung cancer is nearly 20 times the risk in nonsmokers.

The risk of having lung cancer and other cancers can be reduced by quitting. The risk of lung cancer is less in people who quit smoking than in people who continue to smoke the same number of cigarettes per day, and the risk decreases as the number of years since quitting increases.

| *"Both the chemical constituents of tobacco smoke and the numbers of smoking-related deaths are overstated."*

The Health Risks of Smoking Have Been Exaggerated

Eric Boyd

According to Eric Boyd in the following viewpoint, anti-smoking activists misrepresent research to make smoking seem more dangerous than it is. For example, he argues that many of the chemicals found in cigarette smoke, such as lead and arsenic, are found in much higher concentrations in so-called healthy foods, such as wine and fish. Furthermore, Boyd contends that cigarette opponents fail to acknowledge the role smoking has had on reducing the incidence of Alzheimer's and Parkinson's disease. Boyd is a contributor to the *United Pro-Choice Smokers' Rights Newsletter*, a publication dedicated to preserving an individual's right to smoke.

As you read, consider the following questions:
1. What are three fruits and vegetables that, according to Boyd, contain carcinogens?
2. As cited by Boyd, what effect did smoking have on obesity, depression, and breast cancer in Rosalind Marimont and Robert A. Levy's study?
3. According to the author, how will society's irrational fear of smoking affect schoolchildren?

Too much is made of the 4,000 chemicals in tobacco smoke. We're told these chemicals are so harmful that they are responsible for the deaths of millions worldwide. Untold in this "war on tobacco" is that each of the plants we consume consists of an equally daunting thousands of chemicals, many of which are recognized poisons or suspected cancer-causing agents.

Chemicals in "Healthy" Food

Cayenne peppers, carrots and strawberries each contain six suspected carcinogens; onions, grapefruit and tomato each contain five—some the same as the seven suspected carcinogens found in tobacco.

High-heat cooking creates yet more dietary carcinogens from otherwise harmless chemical constituents.

Sure, these plant chemicals are measured in infinitesimal amounts. An independent study calculated 222,000 smoking cigarettes would be needed to reach unacceptable levels of benzo(a)pyrene. One million smoking cigarettes would be needed to produce unacceptable levels of toluene. To reach these estimated danger levels, the cigarettes must be smoked simultaneously and completely in a sealed 20-square-foot room with a nine-foot ceiling.

Many other chemicals in tobacco smoke can also be found in normal diets. Smoking 3,000 packages of cigarettes would supply the same amount of arsenic as a nutritious 200 gram serving of sole.

Half a bottle of now healthy wine can supply 32 times the amount of lead as one pack of cigarettes. The same amount of cadmium obtained from smoking eight packs of cigarettes can be enjoyed in half a pound of crab.

That's one problem with the anti-smoking crusade. The risks of smoking are greatly exaggerated. So are the costs.

Disturbing Flaws

An in-depth analysis of 400,000 U.S. smoking-related deaths by National Institute of Health mathematician Rosalind Marimont and senior fellow in constitutional studies at the Cato Institute Robert Levy identified a disturbing number of flaws in the methodology used to estimate these deaths.

Incorrectly classifying some diseases as smoking-related and choosing the wrong standard of comparison each overstated deaths by more than 65 per cent.

Failure to control for confounding variables such as diet and exercise turned estimates more into a computerized shell game than reliable estimates of deaths.

Marimont and Levy also found no adjustments were made to the costs of smoking resulting from the benefits of smoking—reduced Alzheimer's and Parkinson's disease, less obesity, depression and breast cancer.

If it were possible to estimate 45,000 smoking-related Canadian deaths as some health activists imagine—and Marimont, Levy and other respected researchers think it is not—then applying an identical methodology to other lifestyle choices would yield 57,000 Canadian deaths due to lack of exercise and 73,000 Canadian deaths blamed on poor diets.

Lack of Evidence

There is no credible evidence that 400,000 deaths per year—or any number remotely close to 400,000—are caused by tobacco. Nor has that estimate been adjusted for the positive effects of smoking—less obesity, colitis, depression, Alzheimer's disease, Parkinson's disease and, for some women, a lower incidence of breast cancer. The actual damage from smoking is neither known nor knowable with precision. Responsible statisticians agree that it is impossible to attribute causation to a single variable, like tobacco, when there are multiple causal factors that are correlated with one another. The damage from cigarettes is far less than it is made out to be.

Robert A. Levy and Rosalind B. Marimont, *Regulation*, Fall 1998.

If both the chemical constituents of tobacco smoke and the numbers of smoking-related deaths are overstated—and clearly they are—how can we trust the claim that tobacco smoke is harmful to non-smokers?

The Myth of Secondhand Smoke

The 1993 bellwether study by the Environmental Protection Agency that selectively combined the results of a number of previous studies and found a small increase in lung cancer risk in those exposed to environmental tobacco smoke has been roundly criticized as severely flawed by fellow researchers and ultimately found invalid in a court of law.

In 1998, the World Health Organization reported a small, but not statistically significant, increase in the risk of lung cancer in non-smoking women married to smokers.

Despite these invalidating deficiencies, the Environmental Protection Agency and World Health Organization both concluded tobacco smoke causes lung cancer in non-smokers.

One wonders whether the same conclusions would have been announced if scientific fraud were a criminal offence.

Subjective Interpretations

When confronted with the scientific uncertainty, the inconsistency of results and the incredible misrepresentation of present-day knowledge, those seeking to abolish tobacco invoke a radical interpretation of the Precautionary Principle: "Where potential adverse effects are not fully understood, the activity should not proceed."

This unreasonable exploitation of the ever-present risks of living infiltrates our schools to indoctrinate trusting and eager minds with the irrational fears of today. Instead of opening minds to the wondrous complexities of living, it opens the door to peer ridicule and intolerance while cultivating the trendy cynics of tomorrow.

If we continue down this dangerous path of control and prohibition based on an unreliable or remote chance of harm, how many personal freedoms will remain seven generations from now?

"Given the rate Americans are dying, we'd better start treating obesity like an infectious epidemic."

Obesity Is a Serious Health Problem

Tom Farley and Deborah Cohen

According to Tom Farley and Deborah Cohen in the following viewpoint, Americans are fatter today than ever before. Obesity, the authors note, is associated with heart disease, high blood pressure, and diabetes, among other health problems. For more than fifty years, health experts have admonished Americans to eat less and exercise more, but, in the authors' opinion, these efforts have failed. To reduce the problem of obesity, Farley and Cohen contend, Americans must decrease the availability of junk food and make inexpensive fruits and vegetables easily accessible. Moreover, public policy leaders must work to increase the number of sidewalks and bike paths to encourage people to walk or cycle rather than drive. Farley is a professor at the Tulane University School of Public Health and Medicine, and Cohen is a senior national scientist at the RAND Corporation, a nonprofit public policy institution.

As you read, consider the following questions:
1. According to Farley and Cohen, what hormone helps regulate appetite and physical activity?
2. Why do the authors consider obesity "permanent damage"?
3. What do Farley and Cohen mean by a "Twinkie Tax"?

Tom Farley and Deborah Cohen, "Fixing a Fat Nation: Why Diets and Gyms Won't Save the Obesity Epidemic," *Washington Monthly*, December 2001. Copyright © 2001 by *Washington Monthly*. Reproduced by permission.

O n a Tuesday evening, in a brightly lit classroom at West Jefferson Medical Center in suburban New Orleans, 10 fat people are gathered for their weekly support meeting under the guidance of a physician, a psychologist, and a dietician. One by one, the participants share their successes and lapses. "I lost one pound since last week," says Robert. The group answers with polite applause. Next, Tiffany: "My weight was the same." Sympathetic nods. "But I bought a new skirt and I went down three skirt sizes." Enthusiastic clapping.

The Obesity Epidemic

Behavioral-modification programs like this one designed to treat obesity can be found across the United States. But the participants in this case are children, some as young as five. The average participant enters the clinic at an astonishing 69 pounds overweight. These children are far from unusual. As of the early 1990s, the National Center for Health Statistics (NCHS) found that 11 percent of children between six and 17 were overweight, twice the comparable percentage a decade earlier. Today there are 5.4 million overweight American children, and another 7 million considered "at risk" of joining them.

The epidemic of childhood obesity is only the latest grim chapter of a burgeoning American tragedy. The NCHS found that the proportion of obese adults increased by two-thirds in the 30 years from the early 1960s to the early 1990s. Telephone surveys by the Centers for Disease Control (CDC) have shown obesity rates skyrocketing another two-thirds since then.

In 1991, when the epidemic was less intense, researchers from St. Luke's/Roosevelt Hospital in New York estimated that obesity killed 325,000 Americans a year—eight times the number who die of AIDS, and more than the combined deaths from alcohol, drugs, firearms, and motor vehicles. It approaches the 430,000 per year killed by smoking. But while smoking rates are going down, obesity rates are accelerating. Soon—if it hasn't happened already—obesity will become the number-one killer in America. The cost of caring for those sickened with entirely preventable obesity-related illnesses tops $70 billion per year, about half of which is paid by government.

Losing the Battle

Now, here's the scary part: Everything the medical community has prescribed to fight obesity has failed. Even the best programs, like the kids' clinic in New Orleans, do little more over the long term than keep off a few pounds. Since the 1950s, health experts have been warning Americans to lose weight and telling them how: by eating less and exercising more. Over that time, obesity rates tripled. It's about time we admitted that we are losing the battle against obesity.

This isn't news. Individually, we beat ourselves up for lack of willpower or for choosing a night at a burger joint with the kids over a trip to the gym, dramatizing personal failure even though in today's junk-food-laden society, it's nearly impossible to stay thin. The desk job, the television, the Internet, suburban housing developments and their roads to nowhere all conspire against us. Yet we still view obesity as an individual problem, and so does the government.

But the epidemic is spreading at such an alarming rate that it can no more be viewed as an individual failing than 19th-century cholera epidemics could be blamed on poor personal hygiene. Indeed, given the rate Americans are dying, we'd better start treating obesity like an infectious epidemic. Combating obesity and its many attendant illnesses will not require more cholesterol-lowering drugs or even diet books or workout videos, but rather a retooling of our environment to get us moving again and to put the doughnuts a little farther out of reach.

The Dangers of Midmanagement Spread

Obesity is not just an image problem. Those who are overweight are more likely than thin people to die from heart disease. They have higher blood pressure and greater risk of stroke and kidney failure caused by hypertension; colon, breast, and prostate cancer; gallstones and arthritis. To this list, the National Institutes of Health (NIH) adds "complications of pregnancy, menstrual irregularities, hirsutism, stress incontinence, and psychological disorders (depression)."

Overweight people are also much more likely to develop diabetes, an increase in blood sugar derived from the body's resistance to the hormone insulin, which itself increases the risk of heart disease, stroke, and kidney failure. By damaging circulation in blood vessels, diabetes can lead to infections of the extremities, usually the feet, necessitating amputations. It causes blindness. From 1958 to 1998, the percent of American adults diagnosed with diabetes increased sixfold. At least 20 million Americans now have diabetes, including millions who are unaware. Related medical care costs, currently $44 billion a year, are rising fast.

These days, it isn't hard to spot truly gargantuan people. Watching a 300- or 400-pounder lumber down a supermarket aisle or struggle into an airplane seat, it's easy—perhaps even comforting—to decide that our own 20- or 30-pound inner tubes are nothing to worry about. But because there are so many more of us than them, far more of those who die unnecessarily are in our group. The epidemic isn't just a problem of the grossly obese; it's a problem for all of us.

Americans know that fat is bad for us. We've been hearing it for a half a century, from American Heart Association warnings in the 1950s to pamphlets distributed by the President's Council on Physical Fitness under Lyndon Johnson in the 1960s, to grave CDC warnings about the deepening problem in the 1990s. For a time, in the 1970s, it appeared as though the nation might overcome its fat problem. After Frank Shorter took the gold medal in the marathon in the 1972 Munich Olympics, road races sprouted up everywhere, some with tens of thousands of runners. Sports like tennis and golf also boomed. By 1978, *U.S. News & World Report* was trumpeting a "fitness mania." "We believe that America is going through a physical-fitness renaissance that can make a real dent in degenerative diseases," Richard Keelor of the President's Council on Physical Fitness said at the time. But it was about this time that already rising obesity rates started to skyrocket.

A Coke a Day Makes the Fat Genes Play

Why are we so much fatter than our parents 30 years ago? After all, while dietary surveys over the last 20 years show inconsistent results, none show big increases in the number of calories American adults eat per day. Sports clubs, gyms, and road races seem to be springing up on every corner, at least providing the illusion that some people are working out more than they used to.

NIH researchers are spending tens of millions studying the biology behind this conundrum. They've unearthed some interesting facts: Some people are more prone to become obese than others, and to some extent this bad luck is in their genes. The recently discovered hormone leptin helps regulate appetite and physical activity; a handful of people become obese for lack of an adequate supply. But human genes and metabolism don't trump the basic laws of metabolics: We gain weight when we eat more fuel than we burn. If we eat 2,200 calories a day and burn 2,000, our bodies—programmed for the near-starvation conditions of our hunter-gatherer days—store fat for the next famine. We tend to eat a fairly consistent amount of food no matter how many calories we need, so high-fat calorie-dense foods make us fat.

Laboratory rats switched from rat chow to a "supermarket diet" similar to the high-fat diets of modern Americans quickly grow obese. And, when we're not hungry, we can still be tempted by foods or drinks that meet our biologic cravings for sweet or high-fat foods.

It doesn't take much caloric imbalance to make people obese, only consistency. For instance, if a person drives instead of walks for only 20 minutes every day for a year he will store about 26,000 calories, thus gaining about five pounds. Researchers at the University of Minnesota estimated that over a year, those who spend only five minutes each workday sending e-mails to coworkers instead of visiting their offices will gain an extra pound. Drinking a single can of Coke every other day will contribute enough calories to add about four pounds. Most of us gain weight this way, a few grams a day, a few pounds a year—but enough to shorten our lives.

Fat Failures

As a nation, what have we done to respond to this epidemic that kills 325,000 people a year?

Well, we've spent heavily on medical treatment. But it's a near complete failure. Most drugs tested as obesity cures have been so dangerous that the FDA has kept them off the market or withdrawn them after approval (most notably Fen-Phen). The effectiveness of weight-loss drugs is, in the NIH's cautious word, "modest"; they may cut five or 10 pounds. Intestinal bypass (or "bariatric") surgery can cause fat to melt away, but it's so radical and dangerous that doctors reserve it only for the 300-pound-and-above crowd.

Diets and exercise programs aren't much better. An expert panel at NIH concluded that people who follow strict low-calorie diets can lower their weight by about 8 percent over six months. The trouble is, they gain half of it back within the next two to three years. On average, obese people on a prescribed exercise program only lose 2.5 percent of their weight. And these slim successes are people in intensive programs constantly monitored, educated, and encouraged. Sad as it is to say, we ought to consider obesity, like most other chronic health conditions, as pretty much permanent damage.

If fat people and their doctors can't cure obesity, as a nation we ought to prevent it. Health experts have been trying to prevent obesity for decades. But careful large-scale community trials have proven education programs to prevent obesity to be a complete flop; intervention groups gain as much weight as "control" groups. School-based education programs to prevent obesity do no better (unless they include a supervised exercise component).

Limits to Willpower

We shouldn't be surprised that in the United States as a whole, the call, however urgent, to "eat less, exercise more" has failed. There are limits to the summonable willpower of those immersed in an environment that promotes overeating and laziness. The instinct to seek calories and stockpile them for lean times ahead is hard-wired in our genes. (In fact, the few people who truly overcome their body's natural desire to eat have a psychiatric disorder: anorexia nervosa). It may clear our collective conscience to say that obese people can control their habits in eating and exercise, but it won't touch the epidemic.

A key problem is that health experts usually promote dieting and exercise for obese people rather than healthy eating and physical activity for all of us. Obese people are not likely to lose weight through dieting and exercising, but we all would gain less from healthy eating and physical activity.

The only way most Americans are going to get moving is by making activity a daily routine. There may seem to be a lot of joggers out in parks these days, and private workout spas may be booming, but the percentage of Americans that are deliberately exercising seems doomed always to be small. Only about 15 percent of people tell interviewers in national surveys that they work out regularly, a number unchanged since the mid-1980s.

The same generalization applies to diet. Americans try valiantly to lose weight by dieting, but almost no one keeps on a diet for long. The temptations of easily accessible food are too great. We don't need another diet. We need a way to make healthy eating unavoidable.

Snack Attack

After 3 P.M. on weekdays in New Orleans, teenagers wearing plaid school uniforms of Warren Easton High School drift into the Burger King on Canal Street just off campus to order drinks or fries, or just to hang out. Whoppers cost $1.99. A "Value Meal," which includes a Coke and fries, is just $3.39, while packing 1,190 calories, more than half a day's requirement for teenage girls. If you choose to "King Size" your Value Meal (more fries, bigger drink) for 80 cents, you can boost the calories to 1,570.

Next to the Burger King is a McDonald's. And around the corner stands Rally's, another low-cost burger chain. The kids milling around all three make up the restaurant's largest group of customers.

America is larded with high-fat, calorie-dense junk food. Supermarkets devote more shelf space to snacks than to produce. Vending machines sprout up everywhere (including schools). At a New Orleans gas station recently, we discovered Coke vending machines on every pump island so that drivers didn't even have to walk to the cashier for 140 calories of dissolved sugar. The Coca-Cola company admits its goal is to put a Coke within arm's reach of as many people in the world as possible.

Besides in-your-face availability, these forces include saturation advertising. According to *Advertising Age*, food industry ad spending runs about $10 billion per year. McDonald's alone spends more than $1 billion and Coke more than $800 million. These investments pay off, overwhelming healthy messages like the national 5-A-Day fruit-and-vegetable campaign, funded annually at a paltry $2 million.

The promotion and availability of junk food is cutting down on meals eaten at home (which tend to be relatively healthy) and replacing them with constant snacking away from home. Between 1970 and 1995, the percentage of Americans' total meal dollars spent this way nearly doubled to 40 percent. Between 1977 and 1995, the percentage of meals eaten at fast-food restaurants tripled. Vending-machine snack sales jumped 85 percent in the last three decades after adjustment for inflation. As of 1996, teenagers got 25 percent of their calories from snacks. From the late 1970s to the mid-1990s, consumption of soft drinks increased 131 percent. Americans now guzzle an average of 44 gallons of soft drinks per year—well over one 12-oz can a day for every American, easily enough to add a few pounds to each of us every year.

Fat City, USA

[In 2000,] *Physicians Weekly* dubbed Atlanta "Fat City USA," after its citizens logged a staggering 100-percent increase in aggregate fatness over the previous seven years. Southern food has always clung to the waistline, but it can't account for all of the gain. Other environmental factors had to be at work. Atlanta, of course, embodies all of the worst elements of American sprawl, such as strip malls of big-box warehouse stores with acres of parking lots, six-lane roadways impossible to cross on foot, an absence of efficient public transportation—all of which make for sedentary living. But much of what ails Atlanta can be found in practically every American community.

Americans don't walk any more. If we want to move, we drive. Neighborhoods are segregated from commercial and industrial areas, and sidewalks and crosswalks have disappeared, making it impossible for most of us to walk to a store or to work. In 1995, the National Personal Transportation Survey showed that people traveled on foot or on bicycles for a pitiful 5 percent of trips, down from 7 percent in 1990 and 9 percent in 1983.

Nor are cars the only culprit. Nielsen surveys now show Americans watching an average of four hours of television a day. When we watch television, our bodies downshift into semi-comatose mode, heart rate and muscle activity dropping virtually to sleeping levels. (Thanks to remote control, we don't even get the tiny boost of getting off the couch.)

The Impact of Modern Society on Increased Inactivity

Location or Type of Activity	Effect of Modernization	Impact on Obesity
Transportation	Rise in car ownership.	Decrease in walking or cycling.
	Increase in driving shorter distances.	
At Home	Increase in the use of modern appliances (e.g., microwaves, dishwashers, washing machines, vacuum cleaners).	Decrease in manual labor. Increase in consumption of convenience foods that contribute to obesity
	Increase in ready-made foods and ingredients for cooking.	Decrease in time spent on more active recreational pursuits.
	Increase in television viewing, and computer and video game use.	
In the Work Place	Increase in sedentary occupational lifestyles due to technology—increase in computerization.	Decrease in physically demanding manual labor
Public Places	Increase in the use of elevators, escalators and automatic doors.	Decrease in daily physical activity patterns such as climbing stairs.
Urban Residency	Increase in crime in urban areas.	Prevents women, children and elderly from going out alone for exercise and leisure activities.

American Obesity Association, 2002.

Even simply sitting and talking with friends burns about 35 calories more per hour than watching TV. Just three hours of TV a day can increase an average couch potato's weight by as much as seven pounds a year. Television-watching has even been the subject of the gold standard of medical evaluations: the randomized controlled trial. Over just six months, growing elementary-school children who kept their TVs gained significantly more weight than children who were asked to give them up.

Schools used to make up for these problems at home by forcing kids to exercise in physical education classes. But of the children in the New Orleans obesity clinic, only two said they had PE classes more than one day per week. National surveys showed that the percentage of high schoolers who attended PE classes five days a week decreased from 42 percent in 1991 to 15 percent in 1996; in any given week 79 percent of adolescents do not get PE at all.

All these factors, bad enough for the middle class, turn toxic for the poor and minorities. In poor neighborhoods in New Orleans it is hard to avoid corner stores selling dough-nuts, potato chips, or fried chicken, while genuine grocery stores are lacking. And in poor neighborhoods, responsible mothers worried about the dangers of the streets corral their children indoors, tethering them to television sets and video games. In a Yankelovich Partners survey, nearly one-third of Americans with incomes below $15,000 per year said they did not walk or jog in their neighborhood for fear of crime, double the proportion of those making $25,000. As a result, today, more than half of poor black women are classified as obese.

The Twinkie Tax

Given the overwhelming forces working to undermine our fat consciousness, we might conclude that obesity is inevitable. But there are plenty of things we can do to blunt the epidemic.

First, on the intake side: We can't ban junk food, but we can regulate it. Michael Jacobson of the Center for Science in the Public Interest and Kelly Brownell of Yale University have proposed slapping a tax on soft drinks and junk food. Such a "Twinkie Tax" may at first seem crazy, but even cigarette sales go down when they are taxed, and tobacco is an addictive drug for which its addicts have few alternatives.

A portion of the revenue of such a tax could be used to advertise healthy food or for counter-advertising junk food. One survey found that 45 percent of adults would support junk-food taxes if the revenues went to health education programs. Jacobson and Brownell estimate that even so tiny a tax as 1 cent per can of soft drink would generate $1.5 billion per year. If only one-third of this were used for counter-advertising, it would still only be 5 percent of the $10 billion spent on advertising by the U.S. food industry. But counter-advertising works. When Congress's "Fairness Doctrine" gave us heavy counter-advertising against smoking in the 1960s, cigarette sales fell so quickly that the tobacco companies agreed to eliminate their TV advertising just to get the other ads off the air.

Some of the Twinkie-Tax proceeds could be used to subsidize such healthy foods as fruits and vegetables. Researchers at the University of Minnesota found that cutting the price of low-fat foods in vending machines by 10 percent increased sales by nine percent; bigger discounts correlated with even greater relative sales increases.

We also ought to think about regulating food industry advertising itself. At the very least, we should ban advertising of junk foods to kids, particularly during peak hours of children's television programming. (Parents would likely be eternally grateful to any politician who made this happen.)

Besides taxing junk food and banning its advertising to kids, we can limit the places in which it is available. No one will tell Burger King that it can't run its business, but in the middle of a killer epidemic is it really a good idea to have three fast-food joints within a half a block of a high school? There is no reason we can't, through zoning and planning, regulate the location, density, or hours of junk-food outlets, especially around schools. We also ought to put limits on the location and number of snack-food and soft-drink vending machines. . . .

Let Them Eat Cake

None of these ideas is new. Some health experts have been calling for environmental changes like these for over a quarter of a century. So why haven't we done anything yet? The government agency which ought to take the lead in responding to a public health crisis is the Department of Health and Human Services, but it has delegated the problem to NIH and CDC. NIH is still working on medical approaches: A review of their research grants on obesity showed that 75 percent were for genetic and metabolic studies, and less than one percent was for studies on environmental causes. CDC has done an excellent job tracking the epidemic and publicizing it, but it is not a regulatory agency and can't change government policy.

The federal government's lead agency for nutrition is the U.S. Department of Agriculture, whose primary mission of promoting agriculture often conflicts directly with health goals of reducing food consumption.

Then there's our cherished individual freedom. Some of our fierce individualism spills over into a vague feeling among eminently reasonable Americans that the government shouldn't be telling its people where they can or can't put a vending machine, and also translates into the sense that health is an individual responsibility. But history has shown that in dealing with epidemics of all sorts, ultimately collective, not individual, action radically improves public health.

About 150 years ago, Americans were dying from old-fashioned infectious-disease epidemics. Between 1813 and 1850 in Boston, Philadelphia, New York, and New Orleans, death rates increased by 42 percent thanks to such burdens of newly industrializing cities as crowding, dirty water, and open sewers. Cholera epidemics killed people by the tens of thousands.

The age's medical experts didn't actually know much about the causes of such diseases or how to fight epidemics. But noticing that poor immigrants in the filthy slums of port cities like Boston and New York were particularly likely to get sick and die, they concluded that their eating and drinking habits were "intemperate"; that, as public health historian John Duffy writes, "the basic problem with the poor lay in their lack of moral fiber." The poor had no one but themselves to blame for their diseases. They needed to be taught a combination of personal hygiene and resistance to sin.

It was a nice idea—not so different from today's health gurus' admonitions to lay off the French fries. Of course, like our current crop of self-help dieting books, the personal-hygiene lectures didn't do anything to stop the spread of disease. Then in 1842, a British reformer named Edwin Chadwick published *The Sanitary Conditions of the Labouring Population*, which argued that miserable working and living conditions made the poor sick. They were no different from the rich, he argued, except in their environment. He called for local governments to take responsibility for fixing these problems, ensuring clean water, building sanitary sewers, removing animal carcasses, and providing decent housing.

Chadwick's ideas soon crossed the Atlantic and combined with citizen demands for clean water to create a "sanitary revolution" in the U.S. in the latter half of the 19th century, which forced cities to build water and sewage systems and brought about improvements in housing and working conditions. The revolution virtually eliminated infectious disease epidemics; between 1850 and 1915, death rates fell by 55 percent. This improvement—sudden and dramatic by historical standards—happened before doctors had any successful treatments for infectious diseases or even understood what caused them.

Afterward, the lesson was clear: Society could save lives not by teaching the dangers of filthy water or personal hygiene, but by improving living conditions so that people— educated or not—would drink clean water. Or as British preventive-medicine specialist Geoffrey Rose put it, "The great public health reforms of the 19th century which led to such dramatic improvements were undertaken for people, rather than by people."

If we really care about ending the biggest epidemic of our era and about saving some of those 325,000 lives lost each year to obesity, we'll have to try the same approach.

| *"It is far more important to be fit than it is to be thin."*

The Health Risks of Obesity Have Been Exaggerated

Glenn Gaesser

In the following viewpoint Glenn Gaesser argues that obesity does not cause many of the health problems commonly associated with being overweight, such as heart disease and high blood pressure. Rather, these diseases are caused by an unhealthy diet and lack of exercise, in Gaesser's opinion. Gaesser maintains that a thin person who rarely exercises and eats high-fat foods is less healthy than an overweight person who exercises regularly and eats plenty of fruits and vegetables. Thus, according to Gaesser, lifestyle, not body fat percentage, determines how healthy a person is. Gaesser is a professor of exercise physiology at the University of Virginia.

As you read, consider the following questions:
1. What is the number one cause of death in the United States, according to the author?
2. As noted by Gaesser, how do low-carbohydrate diets affect cholesterol levels?
3. How does the author define metabolic fitness?

F at. F-a-t. Perhaps no other word in our language is despised as much, nor focused on so intensely. Americans are obsessed about fat—body fat—and how to get rid of it. We have been conditioned to view health and fitness in strictly black (fat) and white (fit) terms: A "fat" body cannot possibly be fit and healthy. This fat-versus-fit dichotomy, made popular in the 1970s with the publication of fitness guru Covert Bailey's *Fit or Fat?*, has become the mantra of many a fitness and health professional. You don't have to read any more than the title to grasp the fundamental message of this perennial best-selling fitness bible: A person is either fit, or fat—but not both.

The implications of this myopic fitness philosophy are obvious: The road to a fitter and healthier body is a very narrow one indeed. In order for a fat person to become fit and healthy, that person must lose weight and become lean. This of course implies that "lean" is inherently good and "fat" is inherently bad. Not only is this lipophobic paradigm overly simplistic, it does not stand up against a substantial amount of medical and scientific evidence.

Obesity–Heart Disease Link Challenged

Take coronary artery disease (atherosclerosis), for example—the number one killer in the United States. Conventional wisdom tells us that obesity itself is a major cause of clogged arteries—the rationale being that more fat on the body equals more fat in the blood stream equals more fat build-up in the arteries. However, most of the studies that have looked at the relationship between body weight (or body fat) and atherosclerosis—via coronary angiography or by direct examination of artery disease at autopsy—find that fat people are no more likely to have clogged arteries than thin people. In some instances results entirely opposite to conventional wisdom are observed. For example, when researchers at the University of Tennessee evaluated coronary angiograms of more than 4,500 men and women, they found that the risk of having a clogged artery actually decreased as body weight increased. In other words, it was the fat men and women who had the cleanest arteries. Although this finding is exceptional, the preponderance of angiography studies of this nature do undermine the notion that obesity inevitably results in clogged arteries.

Furthermore, the findings from angiography studies are consistent with countless autopsy studies—dating back to the middle of this century—of the link between body weight (or body fat) and arterial disease. The large-scale International Atherosclerosis Project, for example, conducted in the late 1950s and early 1960s, concluded after analyzing 23,000 sets of coronary arteries—obtained at autopsy—that no measure of body weight or body fat was related to the degree of coronary vessel disease. The obesity-heart disease link is just not well supported by the scientific and medical literature.

Thinner Is Not Necessarily Healthier

The same could be said for the notion that thin people are healthiest and can expect to live longer than everybody else. Contrary to the prevailing medical mind-set, the "thin-live-longest" studies frequently cited by the more vocal of the anti-fat crusaders are far outnumbered by studies demonstrating that body weight—aside from the extremes—is not really all that strong a predictor of death rates, or overall health for that matter. A 1996 publication by researchers at the National Center for Health Statistics and Cornell University illustrates [this issue] perfectly. After analyzing the results from dozens of published reports on the impact of body weight on death rates, encompassing more than 350,000 men and nearly 250,000 women, the researchers found that moderate obesity (no more than about 50 pounds in excess of the so-called ideal body weight) increased the risk of premature death only slightly in men, and not at all in women, during follow-up periods lasting up to 30 years. In fact, the researchers found that thin men—even within the range recommended by the current U.S. government guidelines—had a risk of premature death equal to that of men who were extremely overweight. The researchers warned in their summary comments that "attention to the health risks of underweight is needed, and body weight recommendations for optimum longevity need to be considered in light of these risks."

Ever since the Metropolitan Life Insurance Company introduced its tables of "ideal" weights in 1942—the company called them "desirable" weights in 1959, and did away altogether with the terms "ideal" and "desirable" in 1983—we have been operating under the weight loss industry-reinforced assumption that weighing more than what the height/weight charts say we should weigh is a sure sign of poor health and greatly increases risk of premature death. However, the majority of body weight-mortality investigations have shown that weighing 20 pounds, or 30 pounds, or even 50 pounds in excess of the height-weight chart recommendations is associated with little, if any, increased risk of an early check-out. For example, the current U.S. government guidelines indicate that a 5'4" woman should weigh between 111 pounds and 146 pounds, and a 5'10" man should weigh between 132 pounds and 174 pounds. According to the 1996 study previously mentioned, a 5'4" woman and 5'10" man could weigh close to 200 pounds before their risk of premature death goes up appreciably (excess body weight seems to be riskier in men than in women). This suggests that there are a great many "overweight" Americans—especially women—who are agonizing unnecessarily about those numbers on the bathroom scale.

So if being a little fatter than average might not be so bad, and being thin (at least for men) might not be so good, what does this say about body weight and health? If the concept of an ideal weight is little more than statistical fiction, should we just chuck the bathroom scale, kick back on the sofa with a bag of chips in one hand and the remote control in the other, and nestle into total couch-potato-hood? Of course not (although chucking the bathroom scale is probably a good idea). It's just that body weight, and even body fat for that matter, do not tell us nearly as much about our health as lifestyle factors, such as exercise and the foods we eat. Consider the following scenario.

Randomly select a few hundred men and women (matched for age and smoking habits) and divide them into two groups based on body fat: lean and fat. Next take each person's blood pressure, draw some blood and determine each person's serum lipid levels, and have each person perform a glucose tolerance test (to get an idea of each person's insulin sensitivity). I guarantee that you will find, on average, higher blood pressures, unhealthier blood lipid profiles, and poorer glucose tolerance/insulin sensitivity in the group of fat men and women.

Does this mean that the higher body fat levels caused the health problems? No. It just means that you are more likely to find these kinds of metabolic disorders in fat men and women. But associations do not prove cause-effect. Just because you are more likely to observe high blood pressure, elevated blood lipids and glucose intolerance in fat persons does not prove body fat is the cause of these health problems, nor does it mean that a fat person has to become lean in order to resolve these health problems. The proof of this assertion is quite straightforward. Get these fat men and women to start an exercise program and eat healthier foods—and see how they do. Numerous research studies have done just that. A few examples are described below.

Correcting Health Problems Without Losing Weight

Results from the Dietary Approaches to Stop Hypertension (DASH) clinical trial, published in the *New England Journal of Medicine* in 1997, proved that blood pressures can be effectively lowered by simple changes in diet, without losing weight. Among 133 men and women with high blood pressure, just eating more fruits and vegetables, and consuming low-fat dairy foods with reduced saturated fat, was sufficient to reduce systolic blood pressure by an average of 11.4 mmHg, and diastolic blood pressure by an average of 5.5 mmHg, within two weeks after changing their diets. The reductions in blood pressures were comparable to those observed with initiation of pharmacotherapy—but without the side-effects which sometimes accompany antihypertensive medications. Most significantly, the blood pressure reductions were achieved without any weight loss.

To prove that it's fat in the diet—and not fat on the body—that is the primary cause of blood lipid abnormalities, such as high cholesterol, researchers at the National Public Health Institute in Helsinki, Finland, placed 54 middle-aged men and women on a low-fat (~24% of total calories) diet for six weeks. Total cholesterol dropped from 263 mg/dl to 201 mg/dl in the men, and from 239 mg/dl to 188 mg/dl in the women. Body weight did decrease modestly, by about 2 pounds. The subjects were then switched back to their usual diet (~39% of total calories from fat) for six weeks. Total cholesterol levels returned to their original levels—despite absolutely no change in body weight—requiring the researchers to conclude that the fat content of the diet, not weight change, was responsible for the changes in cholesterol levels. . . .

Being Fit Is More Important than Being Thin

All this evidence suggests that as far as one's health is concerned, lifestyle is far more important than body weight. This goes for longevity prospects as well, as the ongoing—since 1970—Aerobics Center Longitudinal Study at the Cooper Institute for Aerobics Research, in Dallas, Texas, demonstrates. Data on more than 32,000 men and women indicate that the fittest men and women have the lowest death rates—regardless of what they weigh. In other words, a heavier-than-average person who is physically fit has a better chance of living a long life than does a thin couch potato.

Furthermore, a separate analysis of nearly 10,000 of the men in this study who performed at least two exercise stress tests separated by an average of about 5 years (thereby allowing the researchers to evaluate the impact of changes in physical fitness on subsequent death rates), revealed that improving physical fitness level reduced death rates during the 5+ years of follow-up. Men who were initially classified as unfit (defined as being in the bottom 20% of fitness levels for a given age), but who—via increasing physical activity—improved their fitness level by the second fitness examination, reduced their mortality rate during the subsequent 5+ years of follow-up by 44%. Most significant in terms of the weight debate was the fact that the improved longevity prospects were not at all dependent upon weight loss. Results from the ongoing Harvard Alumni Study provide similar results: Sedentary Harvard alums who increased their level of physical activity experienced a 23% reduction in all-cause mortality rate. Because alums who lost weight were no better off

| Fat Can Be Fit

Just being fat does not signify poor health. In fact, research shows that the health risks once associated with weight may instead be attributable to yo-yo dieting. Because fatness is most often caused by heredity and dieting history, and because 95–98% of all diets fail over three years, it is becoming apparent that remaining at a high, but stable weight and concentrating on personal fitness rather than thinness may be the healthiest way to deal with the propensity to be fat.

We must also consider that in our society, it is very difficult for fat people to stay healthy and become fit. Due to prejudicial medical treatment and harassment by health care professionals, many fat people do not receive adequate preventative health care, and procrastinate seeking treatment when there is a medical problem. In addition, many fat people do not feel comfortable participating in activities that would lead to a greater level of fitness due to social stigma.

People of all sizes can strive for fitness by making sensible food choices, following an exercise program, and getting regular check-ups.

National Association to Advance Fat Acceptance, 2002.

healthwise than those who did not lose weight, the reduction in all-cause death rate observed in the more physically active men was in no way attributable to slimming down.

Health Hazards of Obesity Exaggerated

Despite all this evidence suggesting that lifestyle is far more important than body weight in terms of health, and that it might be more prudent to focus on getting people fit and healthy rather than trying to make them thin, the weight loss industry still barrels along like a runaway freight train. Aside from the cultural obsession with slimness, health professionals have done much to sanctify this quest for a lean body—primarily by fueling a medical rationale for fat phobia: Obesity is a major killer. The most blatant—but unjustified—example of this scare tactic is the widely publicized claim that obesity kills 300,000 Americans every year. Former U.S. surgeon general C. Everett Koop asserted as much when he launched his Shape Up America! campaign in 1994. Since then, this figure has taken on a life of its own, appearing in scientific and medical journals and mentioned repeatedly in the media—each time reminding us of the "fact" that obesity is the second leading cause of preventable death in America.

The problem, however, is that there is absolutely no way to prove this assertion. In fact, the most frequently cited source of this statistic, a 1993 article in the *Journal of the American Medical Association*, shows just how misinterpreted this statistic actually is. The article, titled "Actual Causes of Death in the United States," attributes the 300,000 deaths per year to "diet/activity patterns"—not to obesity. Obesity is a physical trait; diet and physical activity are behaviors. To equate them not only is unjustified, it is absurd. While poor diet and lack of physical activity may lead to obesity, the truth of the matter is that the studies used to generate the 300,000 figure looked at the health impact of poor diet and sedentary lifestyle across the entire weight spectrum, not just among fat persons. [There are a great many less-than-healthy couch potatoes with poor dietary and exercise habits who—via luck of the genes—will never be fat.]

Emphasis on Weight Loss Is Misdirected and Hazardous

I am not advocating that we should be complacent about obesity. It's just that continued focus on weight loss seems counterproductive, and may be quite hazardous to the health of those who continually battle their weight. Each year roughly 70 million Americans—nearly one-fourth of the entire U.S. population—attempt to lose weight, shelling out between $30 billion and $50 billion in the process. But despite our perennial efforts to shed pounds, our waistlines are getting bigger, not smaller. It seems what ever we lose, we gain back—and then some. Not only can this be damaging to our self-esteem and mental health, chronic fluctuations in body weight may also do physical harm. In fact, most of the epidemiological studies on weight loss alone show that weight loss increases risk for premature death, primarily from heart disease. This obviously represents a paradox, because weight loss is thought to improve cardiovascular disease risk factors. But this is not always the case.

One of the most popular weight reducing strategies of the past 35 years, the low-carbohydrate diet, actually raises

cholesterol levels (especially low-density lipoprotein cholesterol) and reduces high-density lipoprotein cholesterol (the
heart-healthy kind) despite weight loss. This suggests that
going on a low-carbohydrate diet may actually increase risk
of atherosclerosis.

Another possible explanation for the paradoxical finding
of weight loss being associated with increased risk of dying
from heart disease is the recent evidence which shows that dieting depletes body reserves of heart-healthy omega-3 fatty
acids, thus raising the possibility that weight loss via calorie
restriction may actually make the body more vulnerable to
atherosclerosis. The researchers who reported these findings
warned that "a subtle but chronic risk state could be established if recurrent dieting depletes omega-3 reserves and intake during maintenance does not allow effective repletion."

Metabolic Fitness: An Alternative Health Paradigm

We need a new approach to health and fitness—one that
places less emphasis on body weight (or body fat) and more
emphasis on healthy metabolism—becoming "metabolically" fit. To achieve "metabolic fitness" does not require
having a lean body, nor does it depend upon having the cardiovascular system of an endurance athlete.

In scientific/medical terms, metabolic fitness can be
defined in terms of how the human body responds to the hormone insulin. "Insulin sensitive" bodies tend to have excellent
glucose tolerance, normal blood pressures, and heart-healthy
blood lipid profiles. Therefore, insulin sensitive people tend
to be at lower risk for type II diabetes and heart disease people
who are "insulin resistant"—a metabolic condition in which
the body's cells (mainly those in skeletal muscle, liver and adipose tissue) don't respond normally to this hormone, and
which ultimately may result in disordered lipid metabolism
and elevated blood pressures. Insulin resistance is associated
with high risk for type II diabetes and heart disease.

Although genes play a role, the major causes of insulin resistance are lack of exercise and consuming a diet high in fat
(especially saturated fat) and refined sugar, and low in
fiber—a description that fits many Americans. Because these

behaviors also promote obesity, the "insulin resistance syndrome" (also known as the "metabolic syndrome") is observed more often in fat people than it is in thin people. But as I have pointed out already, a fat person with the metabolic syndrome does not have to become lean in order to become insulin sensitive (i.e., obesity is not the underlying cause of the syndrome). Also, one does not have to be obese to be insulin resistant. An estimated one-fourth of non-obese men and women in the United States are insulin resistant and don't realize it.

Substantial improvements in insulin sensitivity can be changed in a matter of days or weeks, which explains why dramatic improvements in glucose tolerance, blood pressures, and blood lipids can be observed so quickly after starting an exercise program or eating healthier foods. If we can accept the fact that metabolically fit and healthy bodies can come in all shapes and sizes, then the public health message becomes quite simple: be more physically active and consume a healthier diet.

As for exercise, moderate-to-vigorous activity (heart rate in the range of ~60–75 percent of maximum) for ~20–40 minutes per day on most days of the week is suitable for improving metabolic fitness. Intensity and duration of exercise can be modified to suit individual needs. If time is not a constraint, duration can be emphasized while exercising at the lower end of the intensity range. Just as effective, however, is high-intensity exercise of only 20–30 minutes duration. As for nutrition, the best foods to boost metabolic fitness are those you find primarily near the base of the USDA [United States Department of Agriculture] food guide pyramid: Whole grains, fruits and vegetables, and legumes (beans). These foods have plenty of fiber and have been shown to improve health regardless of weight and independent of weight loss.

The Road to Fitness Is Wide Enough for All

It may seem intuitive that exercising more and eating better will naturally result in weight loss. This generally is true, but with a major caveat. Not everyone will lose weight, and it is virtually impossible to tell how much any one person will lose. Most exercise programs and typical diets, result in a weight loss of no more than 5–10 pounds; the average "overweight" U.S. adult wants to lose 20–30 pounds! This discrepancy between what Americans want and what exercise and healthy eating are able to deliver highlights the fundamental problem with using weight loss or reductions in body fat to judge the success of an exercise program or nutrition plan. Exercise and healthy eating should not be viewed merely as means to an end (weight loss), but rather as having their own intrinsic value. If someone quits an exercise program out of failure to reach a particular weight loss (or reduced body fat) goal, then all the benefits of the exercise are lost as well. And far too many people who start exercise programs don't stay with them. Yo-yo fitness is becoming as common as yo-yo dieting.

In America today millions of men and women (and boys and girls) stigmatized as "too fat" are engaged in a perpetual war with their bodies. Isn't it about time we called a truce? Let's face biological reality. Some people are naturally meant to be thin, some naturally meant to be fat. Exercise and diet can modify our genetic destiny only so much. The human body is not an infinitely malleable mass of calories that can be burned down to any shape and size desired. But that doesn't mean we can't all be as metabolically fit as our lifestyle will allow. In terms of health and longevity, the scientific evidence is abundantly clear: It is far more important to be fit than it is to be thin. Contrary to prevailing dogma, the road to a fitter and healthier body is not so narrow after all.

"Vitamins and minerals . . . can reduce the risk for a multitude of diseases."

Vitamin Supplements Are Beneficial

Jonny Bowden

In the following viewpoint Jonny Bowden argues that the American diet does not supply the essential vitamins and minerals necessary for good health. According to Bowden, vitamin supplements are essential to maintaining good health and avoiding disease. He contends that supplements strengthen the immune system, improve memory and brain function, protect the liver, and reduce the risk of cancer. Bowden is a certified nutrition specialist and the author of *Jonny Bowden's Shape Up!*

As you read, consider the following questions:

1. How does the author define the "minimum wage theory"?
2. What is the major difference between Bowden's Level One Shape Up Supplement Program and his Level Two Shape Up Supplement Program?
3. Why does the author advise against asking a doctor about nutritional information?

I am often asked if I "believe" in vitamins which to me is like asking, "Do you believe in air?" Vitamins and minerals are essential to life. You can choose to "believe" in them or not, but your body won't function properly without them.

What people usually mean when they ask that question is "Do you believe in supplements?" And the answer is, unequivocably, "yes."

Here's why: Supplements are nothing more than a delivery system for nutrients, nutrients that were once abundant in our "factory-specified" diet but are increasingly hard to get in therapeutic and protective amounts from our current food supply. Can you live without them? Of course. You can also live without electricity and indoor plumbing. But now that it's available, why in heaven's name would you want to?

The American Dietetic Association and other conservative forces in the nutrition establishment would have you believe that you can get "all you need from food." Quite frankly, this is preposterous. The belief that you can get all you need from food is rooted in a very outdated view of the term "all you need." A little history will explain why.

The Minimum Wage Theory

In the early part of the twentieth century a Polish chemist named Casimir Funk discovered that the anti-beriberi substance in polished rice was an amine (a nitrogen-containing compound). He proposed that his substance be named a "vital amine" which became shortened to "vitamin." Shortly afterwards, Funk and another researcher named Hopkins put forth the "vitamin deficiency theory of disease," which basically said that the absence of these vital substances caused diseases like scurvy (vitamin C), rickets (vitamin D), beriberi (thiamin) and pellagra (niacin). The RDAs [recommended daily allowances] and other "official" views of what we need in the way of vitamins and minerals continues to be referenced to this concept of "avoiding disease" rather than optimizing health.

I call this the "minimum wage theory" of nutrition. If by "all you need" you're talking about what's needed to prevent scurvy, rickets and the like, I'll concede that we don't need supplements. But I don't see much scurvy and beriberi around anymore. Overwhelming amounts of research have shown that vitamins and minerals in therapeutic dosages can reduce the risk for a multitude of diseases, protect the heart, strengthen the immune system, postpone the symptoms of Alzheimer's disease, decrease blood pressure, help with blood sugar control, reduce the incidence of certain birth defects like neural tube syndrome, improve brain function and memory, reduce the risk of cancer, improve symptoms of premenstrual syndrome, help modulate symptoms from allergies and asthma, help with intestinal dysbiosis and irritable bowel syndrome, protect the liver and reduce stresses from environmental carcinogens. Can you get all you need for this level of optimal health and well-being from food alone?

Well, if you were living on a farm, rotating your crops, growing your own food organically, eating it fresh, hunting and eating wild animals that grazed on grass rather than grains and that you honored and respected as the American Indians did the animals they ate, and if you fished for game fish in fresh, uncontaminated waters and if your level of stress was reduced by half and if you were not exposed to smoke and environmental toxins, and if you didn't drink, use tobacco, eat sugar or refined foods or overuse antibiotics, well then maybe you could. But as my father used to say, "If my grandmother had wheels, she'd be a wagon." The point is that you don't do those things (if you do, please invite me to visit—I want to move to where you live). Even in such an idyllic environment it might be hard to get enough vitamin E to have a therapeutic, protective effect on the heart but on the other hand the heart wouldn't be under the same level of stress so perhaps you wouldn't need the same level of therapeutic protection.

The point is, take your supplements.

The Benefits Are Worth the Effort

Recognizing that people differ widely in their inclination to take pills, even those that are good for them, I've created two different supplement programs. Level One is a basic entry-level supplement program that I would like to suggest that you consider taking as an absolute minimum. Level Two is a more comprehensive program that I believe will benefit just about everyone but requires that you pop a few more pills. In the best of all possible worlds I'd like to see everyone in Shape Up on the Level Two program but I'll settle for Level One for now. I think the health benefits are well worth the [effort].

On a personal note, my wife Cassandra and I take well more than 50 of these a day, so we're used to it. We've made it into something of a morning ritual, so it's not only painless but actually part of something pleasant. It takes about five minutes to prepare some morning green tea with lemon and get the supplements ready for the day. Cassandra usually writes in her journal very early in the morning before going to work at the television studio, while I put our supplements together. We have a few moments together, celebrate the day, thank the universe for our lives and face the adventure that's sure to unfold. It takes only a few minutes and has become something of a self-care routine that sets the tone for the rest of the day. At the very least it creates good energy with which to confront any little stumbling blocks that happen to come up. You can include it in a routine of your own making but I promise you that taking a few high-quality supplements to protect and ensure your health is not that big a deal and you can easily make it into a habit.

The Level One Shape Up Supplement Program

1. A high-quality multimineral formula.

Minerals are easily as important as vitamins and are often overlooked. Although there has been an enormous amount of attention given to calcium, I'm actually much more concerned about magnesium. I believe the best research shows that at least 75 percent of women are deficient in this very important mineral, which is needed not only for bone health but for blood sugar control and a host of other important functions. If you are taking a "calcium-magnesium" formula, it should be in a not less than a 2:1 ratio (at least half as much magnesium as calcium) and I wouldn't even mind a 1:1 ratio. Your multimineral should contain at least 400 mg [milligrams] of magnesium.

2. A high-quality multivitamin formula.

Get the best you can find and afford. No matter what people tell you, there's a huge difference in quality from brand to brand. Why? Products vary with regard to the freshness of the ingredients, the quality of the ingredients (which form of the vitamins and minerals they use), the type and presence of fillers and binders, whether or not the product undergoes rigorous testing (assays) of representative batches for potency and quality (and how often) and how bioavailable and absorbable is the final product. Supplement purchases should be taken seriously—don't just grab something off the supermarket, drugstore or even health food store shelf and assume it's good. There are huge differences among supplements—look for products from companies who know what they're doing and that are committed to quality.

The Experts Weigh In

Drs. Walter Willett and Meir Stampfer of Harvard Medical School and the Harvard School of Public Health . . . advised, based on their research and expertise, that a daily multivitamin "makes sense for most adults" for a variety of reasons. They note that the cost of a multivitamin "is so low—similar to that of about a quarter of a serving of fruit or vegetables—that it is unlikely to displace healthful foods in most persons' budgets." Two other Harvard physicians, Drs. Kathleen Fairfield and Robert Fletcher, also . . . concluded that it would be prudent for most adults to use a multivitamin to reduce the risk of chronic disease and emphasized the reasonable cost of this simple insurance against suboptimal nutrient intakes. Dr. David Heber of the UCLA Center for Human Nutrition recently suggested that consumers think of the "basic four" supplements—a multivitamin, extra vitamin C, extra vitamin E, and calcium—as an integral part of their diets along with the four food groups.

Annette Dickinson, "The Benefits of Nutritional Supplements," Council for Responsible Nutrition, 2002.

It's going to be virtually impossible to get a good dosage of high-quality vitamins and/or minerals in one single pill. Most of the better brands will require that you take several to get the recommended dosage. There really isn't any way around this.

Your multivitamin should contain at least 50 mg of all of the B-complex vitamins which, among other things, have been known to help many people feel more energetic as well as have better appetite control. Your multivitamin must contain at least 400 mcg [micrograms] of folic acid and I would prefer that you get 800 mcg.

3. Fish oil capsules.

You're looking for a combination of two important fatty acids—EPA [eicosapentaenoic acid] and DHA [docosahexaenoic acid].

As an alternative to fish oil capsules you could buy a blended oil that contains the omega-3 fatty acids EPA and DHA in the right combination with an important omega-6 fatty acid called GLA (gammalinolenic acid). GLA is found in evening primrose oil and borage oil and women especially find this a helpful supplement, especially prior to their periods. Three superb blended oils that I especially like are Essential Women by Barlean's Organic Oils, Omega Plus by Omega Nutrition and Udo's Choice by Flora, all widely available at health food stores. A couple of spoonfuls of any of these on a daily basis would be terrific. If you can stand it, cod liver oil is a perfectly good alternative (yes, Grandmother was right after all) but it doesn't contain any GLA.

4. Chromium (400 mcg daily).

This trace mineral is next to impossible to get from a regular diet these days and is vitally important in managing blood sugar levels. Many studies have confirmed its value in a weight loss program and even at much higher dosages it has almost no downside. The chromium picolinate form is the most studied.

The Level Two Shape Up Supplement Program

1. A high-quality multimineral formula with at least 400 mg of magnesium.

2. A high-quality antioxidant formula.

3. B-complex.

Dividing your multiple into two formulas—an antioxidant formula and a B-complex—lets you concentrate on getting maximum antioxidant protection in the first and a full spectrum of high quality, good potency B vitamins in the second, rather than having to rely on getting both in the same formula, as is the case in Level One. The same caveats from Level One apply: Look for 50 mg of each of the Bs and at least 500 mcg (preferably 800 mcg) of folic acid.

4. Chromium (400 mcg daily).

5. Fish oil capsules.

6. Vitamin C (500–3000 mg a day).

All the many documented reasons that you should supplement with this vitamin have been written about elsewhere—they're true.

7. Vitamin E (400 IUs [international units] a day). In the case of vitamin E, it really does make a difference that you get the natural form, which in this case means that on the label it will say, for example, "d-alpha-tocopherol," not the less effective synthetic "dl." Ask for a blend of mixed tocopherols.

8. Digestive enzymes.

For many reasons, most people can benefit from these, despite what the American Dietetic Association may think. Many clinicians feel that there is hardly a chronic ailment that doesn't have a digestive (or leaky gut) component and many adults don't fully digest and absorb some proteins because of a lack of hydrochloric acid and digestive enzymes. It can't hurt and will probably help. . . .

Should I Ask My Doctor About Nutrition and Supplements?

Asking the average doctor for information about nutrition is like asking your accountant for information about tennis. Your accountant might actually be a terrific tennis player— maybe he played in college and spends his weekends on the competitive club circuit—but if this is the case, it's a complete coincidence, and he certainly didn't learn how to play in accounting school.

Don't get me wrong. Some of my best professional friends are doctors. I talk to doctors every day. They are all-around invaluable sources of information. The doctors I speak with are some of the best-informed, most brilliant practitioners of nutritional medicine on the planet and have forgotten more about the clinical use of supplements than most people will ever know. They are particularly expert in knowing the interactions of pharmaceuticals, herbs and supplements and have a unique ability to combine science, intuition, clinical observation and research in the time-honored tradition of empirical—rather than deductive—medicine.

And every one of them will tell you this: everything they learned about nutrition they learned on their own. Every one. There is not an M.D. I know who claims to have learned anything of any use about the above-mentioned subjects in medical school. When it comes to food and nutrition most of them basically learned what your average sixth grader learns in a home economics class. My doctor pals will also be the first to tell you that not only did they learn what they learned outside the general medical education model but they encountered—and still encounter on a daily basis—virulent resistance to their integrative approach by the keepers of the cultish flame that is conventional medicine, aided and abetted by the pharmaceutical companies that have just a bit of a vested interest in keeping drugs and only drugs the treatment of choice for any condition on the planet.

It may be difficult to find an M.D. who knows and accepts the profound role that nutrients have on human health and who knows how to use them therapeutically, but if you find one, it will be worth the time spent looking.

| *"Taking vitamins and food supplements is . . . unnecessary for most of us."*

Vitamin Supplements Are Usually Unnecessary

Colin Brennan

Colin Brennan argues in the following viewpoint that most people who eat a balanced diet do not need to take vitamin supplements. He contends that for most people, eating a lot of fruits and vegetables will provide all the vitamins and minerals necessary to maintain good health. Moreover, he maintains, whole foods provide nutrients that cannot be made into pills, such as phytochemicals. According to Brennan, only people with special needs, such as dieters and athletes, require the added vitamins and minerals found in supplements. Brennan is a medical journalist in London, England.

As you read, consider the following questions:
1. Why must vitamins and minerals come from the diet, according to Brennan?
2. Why does Professor Chong Yong Lee say that "an apple a day keeps the doctor away"?
3. In Brennan's opinion, why should people stay away from megadoses of vitamins?

Over the past few years, what could only be described as 'vitamania' has swept the western world, with up to 40 per cent of the population of some countries popping vitamin or food supplement pills daily.

Undeterred by the occasional warning that it is possible to damage the body by overdosing at the breakfast table, there is a blind determination to seek the elixir of life from little brown bottles costing up to £10 [British pounds] a time.

That we need vitamins is not in dispute. It is not down to modern marketing techniques. Vitamins are a small group of substances that are essential in tiny quantities for growth and development. The crucial point about them is that they cannot be manufactured by the body itself. They must come from our diet.

The thinking behind the pill rather than the food source of vitamins is that if you take them by the handful, then you don't have to bother watching what you eat. You can exist on junk food, have a terrible lifestyle and still be just as healthy as the most self-satisfied, highly exercised, keep-fit fanatic. It is easy to see the attraction of this approach.

Apples and Pills

Other people take a less extreme view and try their best to follow the prevailing health advice. They recognise that they will fall short of the ideal and take vitamins as a kind of insurance policy. They take vitamin C as if it was a religious practice and feel they have adopted the modern equivalent of the old adage: 'an apple a day keeps the doctor away'.

Doctors too thought this was a good idea. After all, apples are a rich source of vitamin C, which builds up the immune system. But when researchers compared the effects of apples and vitamin C tablets, the results were quite startling.

The apples contained many other chemicals other than vitamin C, including flavanoids and polyphenols, which acted as anti-oxidants. These are thought to protect against cancer.

The research carried out at Cornell University, New York, found that eating a small apple (100g) gave an anti-oxidant effect equivalent to taking 1500mg [milligrams] of vitamin C, well above the recommended daily dose of 60–100mg.

One of the study's authors, Professor Chong Yong Lee, said: 'Some of the chemicals we found in apples are known to be anti-allergenic, some are anti-carcinogenic, anti-inflammatory and anti-viral. Now I have a reason to say an apple a day keeps the doctor away.'

Too Much of a Good Thing

What seems to have gotten lost in the enthusiasm [over vitamin supplements] is the fact that too much of a good thing can, indeed, be bad. Growing evidence that high doses of individual nutrients may be harmful prompted the Food and Nutrition Board to establish a new measurement called the tolerable upper intake level (UL): the maximum amount of a vitamin or mineral from your food and supplements combined that's considered safe on a long-term daily basis (for a few nutrients, the UL only refers to supplements). There isn't enough data to calculate exactly how likely you are to have an adverse reaction by consistently going over the UL, and experts say that for most nutrients the odds are extremely low. Still, the dangers are real enough to suggest caution. "Even a single very high dose of vitamin A in certain people could conceivably cause liver abnormalities and birth defects," says Paul Coates, PhD, director of the Office of Dietary Supplements at the National Institutes of Health (NIH). "It's not that everybody who takes high doses of vitamin A is going to get these things. The problem is you don't know who will. There's nothing gained by going above the UL. In fact, it may harm you." [In] January [2002], a Harvard study published in the *Journal of the American Medical Association* showed that postmenopausal women with daily vitamin A intakes of 2,000 micrograms (mcg) or more from food and supplements—the UL is 3,000 mcg—had almost double the risk of hip fracture compared to those who consumed less than 500 mcg. "Taking a vitamin A supplement (usually 5,000 international units [IUs] of retinol) appeared to increase the risk of hip fracture by 40 percent," says lead researcher Diane Feskanich, ScD.

Melissa Gotthardt, *O, The Oprah Magazine*, July 2002.

[In 2000], British researchers in a study at St George's Hospital, London, involving 2500 men aged between 45 and 49, found that eating apples was also linked to better lung function.

Health Versus Wealth

Do we really need to damage our wealth by buying pills to protect our health? Dietitians, nutritionists and other experts are all agreed that apart from small groups of people in special situations, most of us do not need to have vitamins or food supplements. We can get what we need from a balanced diet.

Think before you eat is the best advice around. Common sense is the greatest tool to ensure a good diet. People who never eat dairy products will need calcium. It is better to drink milk and eat cheese for the other things they contain, but if you don't like them, or you have an intolerance of them, or you are afraid they will make you fat, then you have to take calcium in tablet form.

It is very important that teenagers and those in their early 20s have sufficient calcium to protect them from osteoporosis (bone thinning) in later life. No amount of calcium supplements taken in the 40s and 50s will make up for a deficiency of calcium that should have been laid down in youth.

A Good Diet Is Best

Sarah Schenker, a dietitian and spokeperson for the British Nutrition Foundation told [this author]: 'Although some groups of the population do require vitamins and supplements, a healthy diet is the best way to obtain the vitamins and supplements we need.

'One of the most important pieces of advice we can give is to increase your fruit and vegetable consumption. These are the foods that are nutrient rich, vitamin rich and mineral rich. Current advice is to try to have five portions per day. This is quite a tall order and many people don't even have half the recommended quantity.

'It has been discovered that these foods contain far more than the classic vitamins and minerals we all know about. They contain many other plant substances, known as phytochemicals, which can't be put in a bottle or made into a pill.'

When to Pop the Pills

Sarah Schenker went on to detail the groups of people who do need to take vitamins and food supplements.

- Women who are planning to get pregnant or have just become pregnant should take folic acid to help prevent spina bifida.
- Asian women who cover up in black robes and have only a limited exposure to sunlight. They may lack vitamin D and they could take that in supplementary form. This could also apply to housebound people.
- People who are malnourished for any reason. They may have come out of hospital after an illness or haven't been eating well. This group could include people who have been on a restricted diet to lose weight or have difficulty swallowing or eating for medical reasons. Slimmers should think of eating more low calorie fruit and vegetables to avoid possible vitamin deficiencies.
- People who are doing intense training for sport.

Elderly people do not need to take food supplements as a matter of course. There may be reasons that make food supplements necessary: problems eating due to loss of appetite; dental difficulties; problems with swallowing or digestion or because they are housebound. But it is not just because they are old, it is a secondary problem. The undernourished and those in training need only take the most basic and inexpensive multivitamin as a precaution. In common with us all they should think of their diet and make sure it is up to the mark.

Concentrating on single vitamins or areas of nutrition can be a mistake, according to Sarah Schenker. We have to think of our overall health, and this is best promoted through a balanced diet. This should always be tried first.

Possible Dangers

A further reason to try to avoid looking for the magic results of mega doses of vitamins is that they can have toxic effects. Some people think that because some is good, more is better, which is not necessarily the case. This is particularly true with vitamins that are fat soluble like vitamin A and will be stored up in the liver. This can eventually reach toxic levels and can damage the liver. Vitamin C will just be secreted with the urine but it can cause diarrhoea at levels of 2000 mg a day, which is lower than the amount many people take to stave off colds.

Just Unnecessary

Taking vitamins and food supplements is neither good nor bad but unnecessary for most of us. There is a lot to be said for saving the money and splashing out once in a while on a nutritious and delicious well-balanced meal at a ritzy restaurant instead.

Periodical Bibliography

The following articles have been selected to supplement the diverse views presented in this chapter.

Anonymous — "'I Don't Eat Red Meat': A Health Strategy or a Platitude?" *Tufts University Health and Nutrition Letter*, June 2002.

Jim Atkinson — "Why Go to the Doctor? Five Reasons You Should Consider Canceling Your Annual Exam. And We're Fairly Certain That Your Doctor Will Agree," *Esquire*, April 2002.

Katrine Baghurst — "Fruits and Vegetables: Why Is It So Hard to Increase Intakes?" *Nutrition Today*, January/February 2003.

Gabrielle Bauer — "Stress and Consequences," *Chatelaine*, March 2002.

Michael Brickey — "The Extended Life: Four Strategies for Healthy Longevity," *Futurist*, September 2001.

Stephen Byrnes — "The Myths of Vegetarianism," *Ecologist*, July 1999.

Michele Deppe — "Natural Refreshment," *American Fitness*, July/August 2002.

Melissa Gotthardt — "Vitamins: What You Need to Know Now," *O*, July 2002.

Michael G. Marmot — "Improvement of Social Environment to Improve Health," *Lancet*, January 3, 1998.

Trudi Matthews — "Disasters Present Health Challenges," *State Government News*, October 2001.

Michael Maupin — "Wellness Is Water," *Swiss News*, January 2003.

Robert Mordacci and Richard Sobel — "Health: A Comprehensive Concept," *Hastings Center Report*, January/February 1998.

Michelle Mueller — "How Virtual Reality Can Help You: Once Found Only in Science Fiction, Virtual Reality Is Being Used to Help Alleviate Pain, Overcome Fears, and Get People in Better Shape," *Current Health 2*, January 2002.

Kathryn R. O'Sullivan — "Fibre and Its Role in Health and Disease," *International Journal of Food Sciences and Nutrition*, November 1998.

D. Ann Slayton Shiffler — "Body Image," *Los Angeles Magazine*, June 2002.

CHAPTER 2

Are Exercise and Weight Loss Treatments Beneficial?

Chapter Preface

According to the Centers for Disease Control and Prevention, 64 percent of Americans are overweight and 23 percent are obese. Many health experts contend that excess weight can lead to significant health problems. The National Institutes of Health reports, "If you are overweight, you are more likely to develop health problems, such as heart disease, stroke, diabetes, certain types of cancer, gout (joint pain caused by excess uric acid), and gallbladder disease."

In spite of these risks, many Americans find it extremely difficult to maintain a healthy weight. Many well-known diet programs, such as Jenny Craig, Weight Watchers, the Zone Diet, the Atkins Diet, and Slimfast, help people shed pounds. However, 95 percent of dieters who lose weight regain the lost pounds, plus more, within five years. Many of these dieters fall into a pattern of "yo-yo dieting"—repeatedly losing and regaining weight—which some physicians maintain puts undue stress on the body, particularly the heart. Furthermore, cycles of losing and regaining pounds can be extremely frustrating and discouraging to a person trying to reach a healthy weight.

There are many theories explaining why Americans find it so hard to sustain a healthy weight. One of the most accepted explanations holds that once dieters reach their target weight, they stop monitoring their food intake and return to their old eating habits. According to the American Diabetes Association, "These people don't realize that they regain the weight . . . because they never give up the old eating habits that make them fat in the first place." Therefore, most dietitians now recommend that people who wish to lose weight avoid drastic, calorie-slashing diets and adopt a healthy food regimen that they can sustain for the rest of their lives. Such a moderate diet promises slow weight loss of only one or two pounds per week, but people who adopt this plan are much less likely to regain lost weight than people who follow radical diets.

In addition to maintaining a healthy diet, the best way to keep off lost pounds is to exercise. In order to lose weight, a person must expend more calories than he or she consumes.

When dieters start eating normally again, their calorie intake increases, but their calorie expenditure stays the same, and the body stores the excess calories as fat. Exercise, however, increases the body's caloric expenditure, thus reducing the likelihood that the body will accumulate fat. "Some believe [exercise] is even more important than restricting calories," health legislator Susan C. Phillips writes in the *CQ Researcher*, "and those who lose weight through diets have a much better chance at keeping the weight off if they exercise regularly." Regular exercise is essential, not only because it burns calories, but also because it speeds up the body's metabolic rate, both of which combat the accumulation of fat tissue.

Health experts contend that the best weapon against obesity is maintaining a healthy lifestyle, which includes eating a low-fat diet full of fruits and vegetables and exercising regularly. Authors debate other methods of weight control in the following chapter.

"There is little mystery about the physiological and psychological benefits [of exercise]."

Exercise Is Beneficial

JoAnn Manson

Exercise is the key to better physical and psychological health, according to JoAnn Manson in the following viewpoint. Manson contends that exercise is associated with a lower incidence of heart disease, diabetes, and muscle tissue loss in older adults. In addition, Manson notes, exercise improves blood flow to the brain, warding off depression and sharpening cognitive function. Moreover, she reports that even moderate physical activity, such as housekeeping and yard work, has beneficial health effects. Manson is a professor of medicine at Harvard Medical School and chief of preventive medicine at Brigham and Women's Hospital in Boston.

As you read, consider the following questions:

1. According to the author, why is fitness not as simple as the "just do it" slogan?
2. What is the body mass index (BMI), as defined by Manson?
3. In the author's opinion, what is the difference between exercise and physical activity?

JoAnn Manson, "Exercise—Staying Physically Active Is Essential to Good Health," *Harvard Health Letter*, vol. 27, November 2001. Copyright © 2001 by Harvard Health Publications. Reproduced by permission.

Like the advice to eat more fruits or vegetables, or admonitions to stay trim, there is something painfully obvious about telling people about the importance of exercise. Most of us don't need to be persuaded that it is good for us. What we need help with is finding the time and willpower to do it. Doctors could do a better job of talking about it with their patients perhaps, but there is little mystery about the physiological and psychological benefits. Hundreds of supportive studies have been done. Nor did it take complicated research to figure this out. Authors of medical tests in China, India, and Greece wrote about the healthful benefits of exercise and physical activity thousands of years ago. We human beings have been talking about getting more exercise for a long, long time.

Yet it really isn't quite so simple as the sneaker company's "just do it" advertising slogan. What kind of activity "it" should be is as changeable as the coaching is constant. The rationale for exercise, however it is defined, has varied with time and place. In the 1950s and 60s in the United States, the emphasis was on fitness, partly because of Cold War anxieties about American schoolchildren falling behind children elsewhere. Now with those Baby Boomers entering their sixth decade, longevity and healthy old age dominates the discussion. Even if you limit your focus to only what's current, there are some variables: age, other health conditions, and living circumstance—they all have to be factored into the exercise equation. But there are a few basic points to keep in mind as you try to figure out what is best for you.

It Is Not Just About the Heart

In the 1970s, if you got caught up in the jogging craze or started to do aerobics, you probably did so out of some belief that you were doing something to protect your heart. The heart is a muscle, and it made sense to many people that exercise would strengthen a muscle. Plenty of studies confirmed the hunch.

The connection between getting exercise and a reduction in heart disease risk remains as certain today as it was 30 years ago—as long as you don't overdo and ease into strenuous exercise carefully. Indeed, it's clear that the risk associated with lack of cardiovascular fitness is similar to or even greater than notorious health villains like smoking, high cholesterol counts, and high blood pressure.

But now there is a sky-high pile of studies showing exercise has benefits well beyond the corridors of our cardiovascular system. Several studies have shown that exercise is an effective antidepressant. It may help with cognitive decline, keeping you mentally sharp possibly by improving blood flow and oxygen supply to the brain. Over two dozens studies point to a real reduction in colon cancer risk.

The evidence for breast and prostate cancer protection is less promising unfortunately. Even some of the hopeful reports are a bit iffy. For example, Canadian researchers published a study in the August 15, 2001, *American Journal of Epidemiology* that found household- and work-related physical activity level was, in fact, associated with lower breast cancer risk among postmenopausal women. Curiously, there was no protection from recreational activity. And they found no association between physical activity and breast cancer among premenopausal women. The results from prostate cancer studies have similarly mixed [results] and [are] open to alternative interpretations.

Exercise and Diabetes

Regular doses of exercise, however, just might be one answer to the growing diabetes problem in the United States. Two notable studies this year showed just how important it might be to preventing the disease. One was an analysis of Nurses' Health Study data published in the September 13, 2001, *New England Journal of Medicine*. It is not surprising that weight control stood out as perhaps the most important lifestyle factor. The Harvard researchers reported that about 60% of the cases of diabetes among the 85,000 nurses in the study could be traced to excess weight. Excess weight was defined as a body mass index (BMI) of 25 or more. (The BMI is a way of measuring weight that takes into account a person's height. For example, someone who is 5 feet 3 inches tall who weights 141 pounds has a BMI of 25.) Still, regular exercise, in combination with a good diet, can help keep off the pounds so it is an important part of weight control. Even in the absence of weight loss, exercise cut the diabetes risk markedly (24%) in this study. Aside from contributing to weight control, exercise probably helps head off diabetes by "training" muscle cells to utilize the insulin and blood sugar more efficiently.

The Mental and Spiritual Benefits of Exercise

The psychological effects of exercise are not as well researched as the physical ones. But many people find that exercise seems to make a difference in their mental state.

• Inactive people are twice as likely to develop symptoms of depression. Depressed people often feel better when they become more active.

• Exercise has a calming effect on many people. One bout of activity can reduce anxiety for hours. Exercise can also reduce muscle tension.

• People whose activities are limited by health problems such as arthritis or heart disease may find their quality of life improves. Exercise increases their strength and stamina and may help them regain the ability to do everyday tasks and feel better about life.

• Exercise based on performing ritualized postures, such as yoga or tai chi, can teach people to focus and develop mental discipline. It can help put them in touch with their spiritual side.

• For people with overly busy lives, exercise offers a temporary escape. It can provide a break from boring tasks or mental exertion.

• Exercise can be good for your self-esteem.

• It can distract you from pain and worries.

• The brain works best when blood sugar levels are in the normal range. By helping to control blood sugar, exercise may help you think better.

• Exercise can be fun! Many of the things you did for play as a child count as exercise. Dancing fast, walking your dog, bicycling, and gardening all strengthen your heart and lungs.

Shauna S. Roberts, *Diabetes Forecast*, August 2002.

The other key diabetes finding came out in August [2001] when the NIH [National Institutes of Health] stopped a large diabetes prevention study a year early because the results were so clear. Participants randomly assigned to a "lifestyle intervention" reduced their diabetes risk by 58%. The intervention consisted of 30 minutes of physical activity per day—usually walking or biking—and maintaining a weight loss of 7%. This study wasn't designed to tease out the relative importance of exercise, diet, or weight loss. In all likelihood, it is combination of all three that makes the greatest difference.

The Key Is Not Exercise, but Physical Activity

At one level, the difference between the two is just a matter of semantics: physical activity is a conveniently vague and more encompassing term than exercise, which connotes running, swimming, working out at a gym, and so on. On the other hand, the change in emphasis from exercise to physical activity does reflect a genuine shift both in government health policy and the research that underlies it.

It turns out that walking, gardening, doing certain kinds of housework with some vigor, and other kinds of activities that we weren't used to thinking of as exercise are nearly as beneficial as jogging, aerobics, and all the rest. Moreover, health officials are concerned that by setting the bar too high, the get-exercise message turned many Americans off. Daunted by all that Lycra and sweat, more of us chose an angle of repose on a comfy couch.

As a result, a landmark 1996 Surgeon General's report on physical activity and health set a pretty liberal standard for what adults need to do. The report said "significant health benefits can be obtained by including a moderate amount of physical activity (e.g., 30 minutes of brisk walking or raking leaves, 15 minutes of running, or 45 minutes of playing volleyball) on most, if not all, days of the week." How fast is a brisk walk? It is often defined as covering 3.5–4 miles in an hour. Age, however, plays a role here because as we get older our cardiovascular capacity diminishes: the same amount of work uses up more of our heart and lung power. A walking pace like that would be classified as light exercise for a 20-year-old but vigorous exercise for the normal 80-year-old.

To make our lives even easier, some researchers are now reporting that we don't even need to be physically active in 30-minute stretches. Their studies are showing that several

10-minute periods of physical activity per day are just as beneficial as a solid half-hour. This validates all the advice you might have gotten about the value of incorporating activity into everyday routines. It seems that one way to stay healthy is to take the stairs instead of the elevator whenever possible. Park the car in a far corner of the parking lot. Better yet, walk instead of drive.

It is good news that "exercise-lite" is turning out to be good for us. But that doesn't mean all the fun runs and workouts with Jane Fonda videos are useless. By and large, the data show that as the level of activity increases, so do the benefits. But we now know that the health payoffs begin at much lower levels.

Do Not Neglect Strength Training

All the emphasis on physical activity makes perfect sense. But especially for people in their late 70s and 80s, strength training shouldn't be neglected. There is an inexorable decline in the strength of our muscles starting at about age 50. But you don't need to join an expensive gym to do something about this muscle loss. Modified forms of the calisthenics that most of us grew up doing—bent-knee sit-ups, push-ups with your knees on the ground—are a good place to start. Simple arm and squatting-type exercises with a lightweight set of dumbbells also build up muscles.

Some studies have shown that just a couple of months of strength training can reverse two decades of muscle loss. Strength training helps maintain bone density, which is especially important for women but also for men. It seems to help with balance, too. These kind of light workouts won't get you ready for Muscle Beach, but they may help keep you on your feet.

"Exercise is not a long-term solution for depression or anxiety."

Exercise Can Be Psychologically Harmful

Rebecca Prussin, Philip Harvey,
and Theresa Foy DiGeronimo

Rebecca Prussin, Philip Harvey, and Theresa Foy DiGeronimo argue in the following viewpoint that although exercise can be a beneficial treatment for depression and anxiety, it can also result in exercise addiction—an acute form of dependency that negatively affects the patient's personal and professional life. Prussin is an assistant professor of clinical psychiatry at Columbia University in New York; Harvey is the director of clinical research and psychology training at Mt. Sinai School of Medicine in New York; and DiGeronimo is a writer whose books include *Raising a Healthy Athlete*.

As you read, consider the following questions:
1. According to the authors, at what point is the line between effective self-treatment and addiction drawn?
2. Why is it incorrect to assume that more exercise will lead to a better mood, in the authors' opinion?
3. As reported by the authors, in what way does exercise provide short-term solutions to long-term problems?

Rebecca Prussin, Philip Harvey, and Theresa Foy DiGeronimo, *Hooked on Exercise*. New York: Fireside/Parkside, 1992. Copyright © 1992 by Fireside. Reproduced by permission of Simon and Schuster, Inc.

For many people suffering from transient mild to moderate depression or anxiety, the benefits of exercise are substantial enough to recommend it as the treatment of first choice. . . .

It's important to keep in mind, however, that persistent depression or anxiety is not always best treated with exercise alone. Although exercise may provide temporary relief for mild, moderate, and even severe depressed moods, there are many cases when it fails to make the symptoms and problems go away completely. Even in these cases, exercise may provide a temporary benefit. The problem is that symptoms are partially or temporarily reduced but not eliminated. Therefore, because exercise has the potential to reduce symptoms temporarily without effectively eliminating them it also has the potential to create a dependence without providing a cure. . . .

Drawing the Line

Exercise is good therapy for some people with negative mood disorders; for others it is ineffective and even counterproductive. The line between effective self-treatment and addiction is drawn at the point where the depressed or anxious person becomes dependent on exercise while trying to maintain an acceptable degree of mood functioning.

Both dysthymia [chronic depression that is less severe than major depression] and anxiety symptoms affect a person's mood "more often than not." Many people suffering these maladies find that exercise can tip this imbalance and allow them to experience positive feelings (particularly in the self-esteem dimension) more frequently than not. Unfortunately, in many cases the lift generated by exercise is short-lived and the exercise routine must soon be repeated to maintain or regain the mood elevation. Thus, an addictive cycle begins.

Your body develops a tolerance for the amount of exercise that you initially found eased the impact of a mood disorder. Quite naturally, there is a tendency to increase the intensity, duration, and frequency of the exercise program to maintain the same level of benefits. As your body becomes conditioned to expect more intense workouts, the positive effects have the potential to become shorter-lived (sometimes lasting no longer than the time of the actual workout). This is when cravings can develop and you'll find that your exercise routine takes precedence over things that were formerly more important. Once exercise achieves this priority status, your positive moods may become dependent upon a workout.

For a long time, you may feel that the energy and time spent working out is worth all that must be given up for it. It's a trade-off that makes sense as long as the workouts remain less in control of your life than your former misery was. After a while, however, the previously contented exerciser can no longer find the same lift and needs to increase the intensity, duration, or even frequency of the exercise session. Soon the workouts will cause as much distress as the former negative moods and the trade-off will become unacceptable.

Some exercise addicts exercise excessively in the mistaken belief that continuous exercise can prevent the occurrence of future episodes of depression or anxiety. Although there is no evidence that this is possible, it's easy to understand that exercisers might superstitiously cling to their regimens in the belief that they are warding off unpleasant experiences. Certainly if you found that in the past exercise was able to ease the effects of depression or anxiety, you might get caught up in the fear that if you stop exercising you'll risk a return of the problem. And so you'd unknowingly instigate a case of exercise addiction to accommodate this faulty belief.

A Dubious Theory

Some excessive exercisers, especially runners, have heard via the grapevine that intense long-distance running relieves negative moods by giving the body and mind a boost through aerobic-based release of endorphins, opiatelike substances found in the brain that can produce the same euphoric and pain-relieving effects as externally administered opiates. Many excessive exercisers believe there is a linear relationship between amount of exercise, release of endorphins, and degree of depression and anxiety relief. The longer you run, some believe, the greater the mood elevation will be. However, this theory does not hold up scientifically.

New studies have found a simpler relationship between exercise and mood improvement. One research team discovered that both running and nonaerobic activities such as weight lifting, equivalent only to a college physical educa tion class, offer an equivalently marked positive mood change. Apparently it is not the kind or degree of exercise that fosters mood improvement but simply the ability of participants to conceptualize themselves as exercisers. In fact, the extent to which participation actually alters the level of a person's self-esteem and mood is not related to the extent of improved aerobic fitness levels. Thus, harder work doesn't necessarily mean a better mood. When people engage in activity that is socially acceptable and positive, they feel good about themselves just because they do it.

The downside of this discovery is that it makes mood-related exercise addiction a more likely possibility in a wider range of exercise modes than was originally thought. As exercisers of all types can find mood alteration in small doses of almost any physical activity, they may arrive at the faulty conclusion that "If a little is good, a lot will be better." And so they double their exercise time seeking double benefits. Because the positive results can be short-lived, the exercisers may return to the specific activity more and more frequently. They find out too late that, as with other addictive substances and activities, more is not better.

Short-Term Benefits

The problem with using exercise as a means of mood elevation is that its short-term positive effects cloud its overall long-term ineffectiveness. Yes, exercise can relieve the impact of depression and anxiety in many people and leave them relatively free of these mood disorders, but for many others, the positive effects of exercise kick in rapidly but last for no more than an hour. If the severity of the depression or anxiety is significant enough or persistent enough, the negative feelings will reappear as soon as the exercise session is over, or even begin to intrude into the exercise session itself. Thus, repeated frequent doses of intense exercise will be required to reduce the emotional symptoms adequately.

What happens to your mood when you don't get your exercise fix? If you have found that your mood problem is relieved by exercise, you may have increased the duration and frequency of your workouts to gain greater psychological benefits. You may have also found that when you are not exercising your moods are still negative and that you have forfeited a great deal in terms of social, occupational, family, and personal interests in your efforts to treat your mood problem. Most likely, you have learned that exercise is not a long-term solution for depression or anxiety states.

Dull Gym Rats

Exercise addicts conduct secret lives in which they furtively plan how they are going to score their next hit. Their need to work out interferes with their work, and deprives their families of their time. Such obsessional behaviour absorbs energy that might otherwise be deployed in more creative, less narcissistic ways. In short, excessive exercising makes one a very boring person indeed.

Matt Seaton, *Guardian*, September 18, 2002.

Even in the best-case scenario, in which exercise is used successfully to treat negative moods, exercise is not always a complete cure. Research data suggest that exercise has its primary effect on self-esteem or self-image. Thus, exercise may not alleviate the secondary problems, such as insomnia, loss of appetite, or poor concentration. So although some individuals are still suffering to some degree, exercise might keep them from seeking and implementing additional and alternate methods of mood management that, when combined with moderate exercise, have persistently shown positive results. These include medication, psychotherapy, relaxation techniques, and stress-management strategies. By ignoring other avenues of help, some people who are self-treating depression or anxiety with exercise are reducing their chances for a full recovery. This, of course, endangers their capacity for full psychological functioning in the future.

The Exercise Cure

Dan is a thirty-year-old account executive with a large mail-order firm who suffers from an exercise addiction caused by anxiety. A year ago, he sought psychiatric help after his medical internist couldn't find an organic cause for his recurring episodes of muscle aches, general fatigue, dizziness, pounding heart, insomnia, and irritability. He had initially thought that he had a heart condition of some type. But he was eventually diagnosed as having generalized anxiety disorder and began psychotherapy to address his incessant worrying about things that most probably would never happen.

During this time, Dan's wife, too, was eager to help him regain a sense of calm. When she saw him start to show signs of anxiety, she would encourage him to join her in a jog around the lake because she had heard that running was an effective relaxation technique. Initially, Dan was less than enthusiastic about this idea. He had never been much of an athlete; his exercising had been limited to college intramurals and an occasional picnic softball or volleyball game. "I've told you," he'd complain, "that my muscles hurt and that I'm tired and dizzy. You don't understand if you think I should get up and run." But later, Dan's therapist also suggested exercise as a possible source of relief, so Dan gave it a try the next time he found himself falling victim to another round of useless, worrisome thoughts.

After his first few runs around the lake, Dan was delighted to find that for the first time in more than two years he could short-circuit his anxiety attacks with a ten- to twenty-minute run. It was as if someone had handed him a miracle cure. At his next session, Dan explained his new plan of attack to his therapist. "If I run every morning," he reasoned, "I shouldn't have any more problems with anxiety, and hopefully"—he smiled to show he meant no offense—"I won't be seeing you much longer."

The following week, Dan returned to report his progress. "I felt great every day after running before work; now I'm planning to add more distance each day because I figure the longer I run, the more benefit I'll gain. At work I still start to feel lightheaded and tense so I'm thinking about running at lunchtime too. This is great," Dan beamed. "No drugs, no therapy, no problems, *and* I'm getting back into good shape!"

Addicted to Exercise

Eventually, Dan canceled all appointments with his therapist, and the therapist heard nothing more from Dan until seven months later when he called the office after suffering an intense anxiety attack. As the story unfolded, Dan explained that until two weeks earlier he had been running each morning and evening. He used this exercise routine to ward off anxiety and found it so vital to his mental health that he put aside other priorities and obligations he would otherwise have fulfilled in those time periods he now rigidly devoted to exercise.

Dan had developed a tolerance for his original quick runs, so he needed to add additional miles to gain the same physical and mental benefits. He also found himself craving his runs and canceling family and business appointments to satisfy the urge and to calm his fears. Then he fell down a flight of stairs while moving some boxes into the attic. Dan hurt his left knee and couldn't run for at least a month.

Anxiety Symptoms Return

Because Dan's ability to function normally had become dependent on exercise he was now experiencing a return of his anxiety symptoms. His original problem with anxiety gradually returned along with an abrupt onset of difficulties associated with the compounding addiction problems. "I feel so sluggish," he confessed. "I have no appetite; I can't sleep; my head hurts, and I feel useless and angry. What's happening? I feel worse now than I did when I first came to you!" Dan returned to his therapist for an answer to his question and also because he had lost the support of his family and friends who had become tired of coming in second to exercise and didn't want to hear his complaining now that he had to spend more time at home. Dan had temporarily lost the external mechanism that enabled him to feel good about himself. Without exercise, Dan had lost his "cure" for anxiety, his self-esteem, and his ability to function in the manner necessary to his work and personal life.

In moderate amounts, exercise could have helped Dan deal with his problems and given him enough time and objectivity to seek additional forms of help. Unfortunately, Dan, like many others who use exercise to self-treat anxiety or depression, fell hard for the idea that more is better. Now Dan and his therapist had to find a way to help him use alternate types of exercise that could be practiced with a bad knee; Dan had to ease himself into a program that would reduce the frequency of exercise and maintain his self-esteem. Dan and his therapist had to return to the original problem of his mood disorder and start again to look for a way to help him function calmly and happily.

"*Dietary supplement products containing ephedra provide dubious health benefits while posing serious health risks.*"

Ephedra Causes Serious Health Problems

James Guest and Marvin M. Lipman

The following viewpoint is excerpted from a letter from Consumers Union, a nonprofit consumer advocacy organization, to Tommy Thompson, the secretary of the Department of Health and Human Services. The authors, James Guest and Marvin M. Lipman, urge the Federal Drug Administration (FDA) to ban the use of ephedra, an herbal weight loss aid, in all dietary supplements. According to the authors, ephedra causes strokes, heart attacks, seizures, and other serious health complications. FDA regulation is necessary, the authors argue, because ephedra manufacturers routinely suppress reports of health problems by ephedra users. Guest is the president of Consumers Union, and Lipman is Consumers Union's chief medical adviser.

As you read, consider the following questions:

1. Why do reported complaints about ephedra represent the tip of the iceberg, according to the authors?
2. As reported by Guest and Lipman, which nongovernmental associations have banned the use of ephedra?
3. Which action of Twinlab's do the authors support?

For the reasons outlined below, Consumers Union, the nonprofit publisher of *Consumer Reports* magazine, urges the U.S. Food and Drug Administration (FDA) to immediately declare dietary supplement products containing ephedrine alkaloids and ma Huang (collectively referred to as "ephedra" in this letter) to be adulterated under Section 402 of the Federal Food Drug and Cosmetic Act. Since dietary supplement products containing ephedra have been linked to many serious adverse health events, including death, we ask you to declare such products adulterated . . . because they "[present] a significant or unreasonable risk of illness or injury under . . . conditions of use recommended or suggested in labeling." In addition, we urge you to initiate proceedings to ban the production and sale of dietary supplements containing ephedra . . . because they "pose an imminent hazard to public health or safety."

We are also very alarmed by reports that major herbal supplement manufacturers have suppressed adverse event reports related to herbal supplement products. To protect consumer health and safety, we strongly urge you to seek the necessary statutory authority to require mandatory reporting of all adverse event reports received by manufacturers to the FDA, and to require additional label information for consumers to facilitate reporting of adverse reactions to FDA Medwatch.

Reports of Ephedra Risks

Dietary supplement products containing ephedra provide dubious health benefits while posing serious health risks to consumers. From January 1993 through October 2000, the FDA received 1,398 reports of adverse events linked to herbal supplements containing ephedra, including 81 deaths, 32 heart attacks, 62 reports of cardiac arrhythmia, 91 reports of hypertension, 69 strokes and 70 seizures. Complaints about herbal supplements containing ephedra constituted 42% of all dietary supplement complaints, and 59% of all reported deaths.

As you well know, those complaints likely represent only the tip of the iceberg, because the vast majority of adverse reactions to dietary supplements or medications are never reported to the FDA, or indeed, to any health professional or agency.

The American Association of Poison Control Centers has reported a steadily increasing number of serious adverse events related to supplements containing ephedra over the last five years. Recent data released by the AAPCC indicates that in the year 2001 alone there were:

• 812 reported events relating to exposure to dietary supplements containing ephedra as a sole ingredient, including 3 deaths, 103 adverse reactions, 10 "major effects" (defined as exhibiting signs or symptoms that were life-threatening or resulted in significant residual disability) and 139 "moderate effects" (defined as exhibiting symptoms or signs that were more pronounced, more prolonged or more systemic in nature than minor symptoms—and where usually some form of treatment is indicated). Of the 812 exposures, 440 persons (54%) were treated in a health care facility. 48% of reported exposures occurred in individuals over 19 years of age.

• 7,115 reported events linked to exposures to multi-botanical supplements containing ephedra as an ingredient, including 3 deaths, 1,075 adverse reactions, 87 "major effects" and 1,325 "moderate effects." Of the 7,115 exposures, 3,849 persons (54%) were treated in a health care facility. 43% of reported exposures occurred in individuals over 19 years of age.

Compelling Evidence

Two recent independent studies from well-respected academic centers, reported in peer-reviewed journals, scrutinized adverse events reports filed with the FDA between 1995 and 1999. In the reports, researchers found dozens of cases of abnormal heartbeats, strokes and heart attacks that were likely related to ephedra use.

[Researcher D.] Samenuk and others at the New England Medical Center in Boston analyzed almost 1,000 cases of possible ephedra toxicity submitted to the FDA. They reported in [an] issue of *Mayo Clinic Proceedings* that untoward events were clearly related to immediate prior use of the drug in 37 people, and that 36 of these 37 victims had taken the product according to the manufacturer's directions. Sixteen suffered a stroke; 10 had a heart attack; and 11 died. The study concluded that "ma Huang use is temporally related to stroke, myocardial infarction, and sudden death; (2) underlying heart or vascular disease is not a prerequisite for ma Huang-related adverse events; and (3) the cardiovascular toxic effects associated with ma Huang were not limited to massive doses."

In the December 21, 2000 issue of *The New England Journal of Medicine*, [Researchers C.A.] Haller and [N.L.] Benowitz from the University of California in San Francisco analyzed 140 cases of alleged ephedra toxicity that were reported to the FDA from 1997 to 1999. Abnormal heart rhythms, increases in blood pressure, stroke, sudden death, and heart attack led the list. Of those reactions, 62 percent were thought to be "definitely or probably" or "possibly" due to ephedra. Eight of the 10 deaths were attributed to ephedra, including that of a 15-year-old girl.

The few clinical studies that have been done to date are short-term and have used small numbers of subjects. Adverse reactions included elevated blood pressure, palpitations, chest pain, and extreme irritability. Dropout rates were high in the ephedra-using volunteers.

Undisclosed Information

Strong evidence has now emerged that manufacturers of dietary supplements containing ephedra have been concealing substantial numbers of consumer complaints regarding their products:

• On August 15, 2002, the Justice Department disclosed that it was investigating whether Metabolife (a major manufacturer and distributor of ephedra products), had made false statements to the FDA regarding the existence of consumer complaints about its products. On the same day, Metabolife announced that it would turn over 13,000 consumer health complaints or "adverse event reports" to the FDA. After analyzing the Metabolife adverse events reports, the special investigations division of the House Committee on Government Reform concluded that 2,000 of the 13,000 reports were "significant" effects, including three deaths, 20 heart attacks, 24 strokes, 40 seizures, 465 episodes of chest pains

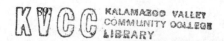

and 966 reports of heart rhythm disturbances.

• Two years ago, depositions in a lawsuit in San Francisco against E'ola (a Utah-based multilevel-marketing firm) regarding a death allegedly linked to ephedra revealed that the company had received 3,500 customer complaints about one of its ephedra weight-loss products. According to the *San Francisco Chronicle*, none of the complaints were ever disclosed to the FDA.

What Evidence Is There That Ephedra May Be Harmful?

• A RAND Corporation study commissioned by NIH [National Institutes of Health] concluded ephedra is associated with higher risks of mild to moderate side effects such as heart palpitations, psychiatric and upper gastrointestinal effects, and symptoms of autonomic hyperactivity such as tremor and insomnia, especially when taken with other stimulants.

• The RAND review of 16,000 adverse event reports revealed two deaths, four heart attacks, nine strokes, one seizure, and five psychiatric cases involving ephedra in which the records appeared thorough and no other contributing factors were identified. RAND called such cases "sentinel events," because they may indicate a safety problem but do not prove that ephedra caused the adverse event.

• A study published [in March 2003] in the *Annals of Internal Medicine* found that although ephedra products make up less than 1 percent of all dietary supplement sales, these products account for 64 percent of adverse events associated with dietary supplements.

• A study published in the journal *Neurology* concluded that the rate of hemorrhagic (bleeding) strokes among ephedra users was statistically significantly higher than among nonusers, for people who take doses above 32 milligrams a day. Many ephedra dietary supplement labels recommend that users take up to approximately 100 mg of ephedra daily.

U.S. Department of Health and Human Services, "Reducing Ephedra-Related Risks," March 4, 2003.

While it isn't clear how many other manufacturers and sellers of ephedra products may be suppressing information regarding potential health effects, those examples do not inspire confidence that serious health impacts arising from the use of herbal supplements will be promptly reported to responsible health authorities under a voluntary reporting system. This also underscores the dangers of allowing herbal medicines in the marketplace without premarket safety testing and a rigorous post-marketing surveillance system. Those are very serious problems that badly need to be addressed by the Congress and the FDA without additional delay.

Taking Action

While the FDA has thus far failed to act to protect the public health from these dangerous products, other entities from Canada and Western Europe, to states and localities across the United States, are working to protect the public from injury and death.

• Canada, the United Kingdom and Germany all prohibit sales of ephedra, while other European countries allow the sale of ephedra products only by prescription. At least ten U.S. states, and several local governments have imposed various restrictions on ephedra sales, such as requiring a prescription, outlawing sales to minors, or limiting the maximum dose.

• The American Medical Association has called for the FDA to remove products containing ephedra from the marketplace.

• The National Collegiate Athletic Association, the International Olympic Committee, and the National Football League have already banned the use of ephedra-containing products.

• According to information recently released by Public Citizen Health Research Group, from 1997 through part of 2001, as many as 33 members of the U.S. military have died in ephedra-related deaths. Those who died were between their early 20s and early 40s and were reportedly in good health. As a result, the Army and Air Force military exchanges have removed such products from military commissary shelves worldwide.

• On November 11, [2002,] Twinlab Corporation, a major herbal supplement manufacturer based in Hauppauge, New York, announced it would stop all sales of products containing ephedra as of March 2003, because of "escalating insurance costs and regulatory uncertainties."

While we believe that other manufacturers should follow Twinlab's lead—and voluntarily remove ephedra products from the marketplace—it's clear that consumers need more than just voluntary action, or even state and local legislation, to be adequately protected. Although some U.S. states and localities, such as California, Westchester County, New York and Huntington, New York have banned the sale of ephedra to under-age purchasers, its hazards are by no means limited to minors. We are particularly concerned about the potential risks to adults who may have known or unknown conditions such as cardiovascular disease, diabetes and hypertension, or who may combine their intake of ephedra with caffeine, other herbal supplements and/or other medications. We are also concerned about the risks to consumers caused by further delay and inaction by the federal government.

Consumers Must Protect Themselves

As a national consumer organization, our position is clear. We believe consumers should immediately stop using products containing ephedra, and educate themselves and others about the serious dangers of these products. Further, we believe consumers should discuss the use of any herbal supplement with their physician prior to taking it, and promptly report any adverse reactions to such products to their physician and to the FDA Medwatch database.

We also believe that the federal government must now act to protect consumers against the known and widely acknowledged hazards of ephedra. Compared to the adverse event data that have accumulated for products containing ephedra, certain prescription drugs have been withdrawn from the market for much less adverse events.

We are very concerned that delay by the FDA in addressing this serious public health hazard continually subjects consumers to unnecessary risk, and undermines public confidence in the government institutions that are charged with protecting consumer health and safety.

It is for the foregoing reasons that we petition the FDA to declare dietary supplements containing ephedrine alkaloids and ma Huang to be adulterated, and to initiate a proceeding to ban the manufacture, sale, introduction, or delivery for introduction into interstate commerce of all such products immediately. We also urge you to seek the necessary statutory authority to require mandatory reporting of all adverse event reports received by manufacturers to the FDA, and to require that all herbal supplement products include label information that directs consumers to report any adverse health effects to their doctor and to FDA's Medwatch.

| *"Ephedra is safe and effective if used responsibly."*

The Health Risks of Ephedra Have Been Exaggerated

Barbara Zeitlin Kravets

According to Barbara Zeitlin Kravets in the following viewpoint, the weight loss supplement ephedra has been unfairly vilified by the media. She argues that ephedra is the most effective weight loss aid available and that its side effects—such as dizziness, headache, or increased blood pressure—are minimal when it is taken correctly. Kravets maintains that taking ephedra responsibly will protect consumers from dangerous side effects and improve ephedra's reputation as a safe weight loss supplement. Kravets is a licensed and board certified clinical nutritionist.

As you read, consider the following questions:
1. Why does Daniel Mowrey contend that ephedra is the most effective weight loss product available, as quoted by Kravets?
2. In the author's opinion, who should not use ephedra?
3. What does Kravets consider common sense advice for ephedra consumers?

How is your weight? Going up, not down? Have you tried diet and exercise? We are so fat in America that it has been called a national emergency. Six out of ten of us are overweight or obese.

And, obesity matters! As a matter of fact, obesity is a greater risk to health than is smoking, heavy drinking, or being poor. No wonder people are reaching for supplements such as ephedra, along with proper nutrition and exercise, to help in the battle of the bulge.

An Insignificant Percentage

More than 12 million Americans take ephedra safely and effectively for weight loss. With the on-going controversy over the diet product Metabolife, it's interesting to note that in approximately 12,000 pages of consumer comments on the product, there were actually only 89 calls alleging significant side effects. This information comes from Steven B. Karch, M.D., assistant medical examiner for San Francisco.

In light of this, it's difficult to understand why [in] summer [2002] Senator Dick Durbin (D-IL), chair of the Senate Governmental Affairs Oversight Subcommittee, called for an immediate determination as to whether dietary supplements such as ephedra constitute an "imminent hazard" to the nation's public health.

Is this a bad rap for a good supplement?

Quite likely it is. After all, *Ephedra sinica*, also known as ma huang, is a plant that has been used for thousands of years in Chinese medicine. Ephedra contains "ephedrine alkaloids" and other alkaloids, which are naturally occurring (as opposed to "pseudo" ephedra alkaloids such as those found in Sudafed).

The Chinese have used ephedra for many reasons, but here in America we use ephedra to help with weight loss. Specifically it's useful for burning fat. Daniel Mowrey, Ph.D., is president of the non-profit American Phytotherapy Research Laboratory, is author of *Fat Management: The Thermogenic Factor*, and is a scientific investigator who's been on the frontline of ephedra research for 12 years. He says, "Ephedra enhances the working of brown adipose tissue (BAT) and other calorie wasting tissue. Ephedra is the only plant material currently known to safely stimulate BAT to burn fat. That makes ephedra the most effective weight loss product we've ever had."

Common Knowledge

Although knowledgeable healthcare providers and millions of American consumers know that ephedra is effective and safe if used responsibly, research studies underscore its safety. Researchers at prestigious Harvard and Columbia Universities have confirmed the safety and effectiveness of ephedra supplements for weight loss in healthy Americans when *used as directed with appropriate serving limits, warnings, and precautions.* Here are their own powerful words about the effect and the safely of ephedra. "In this six-month placebo-controlled trial, herbal ephedra/caffeine (90/192 mg per day) promoted body weight and body fat reduction and improved blood lipids without significant adverse events." This is but one of the numerous studies showing the effectiveness and safety of ephedra when taken responsibly.

Then what is the bad rap for ephedra? It has to do with the side effects. Yes, there are side effects, as there are with other stimulating substances, including coffee. If you misuse, or overuse ephedra, (or coffee) you might experience: nervousness, dizziness, tremor, alternation in blood pressure or heart rate, headache, gastrointestinal distress, chest pain, myocardial infarction, hepatitis, stroke, seizures, psychosis, and death.

That is why herbal manufacturers of ephedra have warnings on their labels. Just as they say on TV, "it is not for everyone." Ephedra should not be used by anyone who is under 18, or pregnant or nursing. An informed healthcare provider should be consulted before using ephedra if you have any of the following: heart disease, thyroid disease, diabetes, high blood pressure, a psychiatric condition, difficulty in urinating, prostate enlargement, or seizure disorder. You should consult a provider if you are using a monoamine oxidase inhibitor (MAOI) or any other prescription drug, or if you are using an over-the-counter drug containing ephedrine, pseudoephedrine or phenylpropanolamine (ingredients found in certain allergy, asthma, cough/cold and weight control products).

Ephedra Is Safe When Taken as Directed

Experts who have reviewed all of the available historical and clinical data agree: You can take Ephedra safely if you stick to the serving limits and follow the warnings and precautions adopted by the Industry.

Industry adopted these standards as a recommendation for distributors, marketers and consumers of dietary supplement products containing ephedrine alkaloids. A panel of experts from a variety of scientific and medical backgrounds endorsed the standards that the trade recommendation established. In addition, several states, including Ohio, Michigan, Nebraska, Texas, Oklahoma, Hawaii, and Washington have adopted portions of these standards as state law.

Although many Ephedra product manufacturers follow the industry recommendation, not all do, so check the label of your Ephedra product to make sure it bears the recommended serving limits and warnings. If information and warnings comparable to those listed in the trade recommendation are not included on the label, then the EEC [Ephedra Education Council] recommends that you do not purchase the product. It is very important that you read product labels, warnings and cautions, and follow the directions. Ephedra is not for everyone and must be used responsibly.

Ephedra Education Council, Ephedrafacts.com, 2003.

The reason the Harvard-Columbia study is so reliable in its results is that study participants were excluded from the study if they had any of the problems stated above. The researchers were smart to do this. They knew what it said on the labels for ephedra. But, there are people who don't read labels and who abuse ephedra, who have not yet figured out how to use ephedra with common sense. Lack of responsible usage of ephedra increases side effects, which alerts government agencies.

The Pros Outweigh the Cons

As Dr. Mowrey and numerous other doctors and scientists have pointed out, the FDA has tried before to get ephedra off the market, but they failed. They failed because at the hearings there were many more pros than cons about ephedra. Dr. Mowrey is now concerned that some medical journals, emphasizing side effects stemming from improper use of the herb, are printing negative opinion articles about it. Studies that shed positive light on the use of ephedra, like the Harvard study, are not printed in conjunction with the negative opinion articles, and Dr. Mowrey's own letter of protest to the editor was ignored. Worse yet, ephedra suffered a bad public relations blow over the Metabolife ephedra product. This came when the president of the company said there were no "Adverse Events Reports" when there were actually many thousands of calls to his company about the product. Even though the overwhelming majority of the calls were about harmless occurrences, the fact that he was not immediately forthcoming shed a very bad light on his product and ephedra in general.

The Ephedra Education Council of the American Herbal Products Association has some good "common sense" legal advice for Senator Dick Durbin and his committee. The Council supports a California consumer protection bill on ephedra that reflects a "common sense" approach, including strict warning labels and a prohibition on sales to minors that have long been supported by the industry. With this bill, consumers will continue to have access to ephedra dietary supplements in all states. Consumers should check products to ensure that recommended serving limits and warnings are included and follow the label warnings carefully.

And, what is good "common sense" advice for the consumer? If you are considering ephedra for weight loss because it is effective, read the label on the box, then consult your doctor. If your doctor is not knowledgeable about ephedra, then find an integrative medical practitioner who is savvy about this subject and follow her instructions. Incorporate a proper diet and exercise. Stay in touch with your health practitioner and report any side effects.

In this way, there will be no bad rap for a good supplement.

Periodical Bibliography

The following articles have been selected to supplement the diverse views presented in this chapter.

Douglas Fox	"Hard Cheese: It's Just Not Fair. All That Gouda and Cheddar You Eat to Keep Your Bones Hard and Strong May Be Having the Opposite Effect," *New Scientist*, December 15, 2001.
Michael Fumento	"Big Fat Fake: The Atkins Diet Controversy and the Sorry State of Science Journalism," *Reason*, March 2003.
Elaine Gavalas	"The Great Diet Debate," *Better Nutrition*, May 2000.
F. Greenway	"The Safety and Efficacy of Pharmaceutical and Herbal Caffeine and Ephedrine Use as a Weight Loss Agent," *Obesity Reviews*, 2001.
Harvard Heart Letter	"Can Drugs Help You Lose Weight?" March 2002.
Harvard Men's Health Watch	"Diet Wars I: How Do You Measure Up?" December 2002.
Unmesh Kher	"How to Sell XXXL: With More Americans Overweight, Smart Firms Aim to Sell Them Things to Make Their Lives More Comfy," *Time*, January 27, 2003.
Kristine Kieswer	"Make Your Genes Fit: Genetic Manipulation Through Nutrition and Exercise May Help Achieve Weight Loss Goals," *American Fitness*, March/April 2002.
Victor M. Parachin	"Why Exercise Is the Best Medicine," *Vibrant Life*, November/December 2001.
Shauna S. Roberts	"Why Exercise Matters: Exercising Does More Than Burn Calories—It Can Also Boost Your Physical, Mental, and Even Financial Wellbeing," *Diabetes Forecast*, August 2002.
Douglas Schar	"Weight Loss Herbs That Work—and They're Safe!" *Prevention*, August 2001.
Matt Seaton	"Confessions of a Fitness Fanatic: Eating Less and Exercising Are Simple Cures for Obesity, but an Addiction to Activity Can Be Just as Unhealthy," *Guardian*, September 18, 2002.

CHAPTER 3

Are Alternative Therapies Beneficial?

Chapter Preface

The *Merriam-Webster Medical Dictionary* defines alternative medicine as "any of various systems of healing or treating disease (as homeopathy, chiropractic, naturopathy, Ayurveda, or faith healing) that are not included in the traditional curricula taught in medical schools of the U.S. and Britain." Alternative therapies have become increasingly popular as more and more people have become dissatisfied with conventional medicine and the impersonal nature of managed care. One of the most controversial alternative therapies, acupuncture, is even beginning to gain support within the medical community.

Acupuncture is an ancient Chinese practice that is based on the belief that the body's vital energy, known as *qi* (pronounced "chee"), circulates through channels, called meridians, that connect to bodily organs and functions. Illness results when disharmonies develop that block the flow of energy through these meridians. Acupuncture involves inserting needles into various points on the body, called acupoints, which is believed to reestablish normal energy flow through these various channels. Enthusiasts maintain that acupuncture helps relieve chronic pain, anxiety, menstrual pain, depression, headaches, and other ailments. Some supporters claim that acupuncture has been successful at helping patients overcome addictions to drugs, including alcohol and tobacco.

Skeptics, however, argue that unproven theories and dubious standards make acupuncture a risky therapy. The National Health Council Against Fraud contends that "[acupuncture's] theory and practice are based on primitive and fanciful concepts of health and disease that bear no relationship to present scientific knowledge." Detractors note that evidence that supports acupuncture's effectiveness relies on practitioners' observations and patients' testimonials rather than on scientifically conducted studies. Moreover, according to psychiatry professor George A. Ulett, questionable licensing standards frequently subject patients to the care of unqualified practitioners. He states, "Certification of acupuncturists is a sham. While a few of those so accredited are naïve physicians, most are nonmedical persons who only play at being doctor and use this certification as an umbrella for a host of unproven New Age hokum treatments." Inexperienced or poorly trained acupuncturists can inflict serious injuries on patients, such as punctured blood vessels and lungs, convulsions, infections from unsterile needles, and nerve damage.

Despite these risks, some medical professionals are embracing acupuncture as an effective treatment for pain. Supporters contend that the needles stimulate the release of endorphins, a neurotransmitter that reduces pain. According to experts, numerous studies over the past twenty years have shown that inserting needles into acupoints stimulates nerves in the underlying muscles. That stimulation, researchers believe, sends impulses up the spinal cord to the brain. Somehow those impulses lead to the release of endorphins and monoamines, chemicals that block pain signals in the spinal cord and the brain. In 1997 the National Institutes of Health announced that there was sufficient evidence of acupuncture's effectiveness to warrant further research by the medical community. According to spokesman David J. Ramsay, "We need more high quality research to validate what appears to be useful for the millions of Americans that have used acupuncture in [the United States]. The challenge in studying acupuncture is to integrate the theory of Chinese medicine into the conventional Western biomedical research model and into the conventional health care arena."

Whether acupuncture will be integrated into conventional medicine remains to be seen. In the meantime, skeptics advise patients to thoroughly investigate the qualifications of acupuncturists before submitting to their care. Authors discuss other alternative therapies in the following chapter.

"Doctors . . . are using acupuncture and herbs as well as surgery, medication, and exercise to help rehabilitate patients."

Alternative Therapies Are Beneficial

Susan Ince

According to Susan Ince in the following viewpoint, certain alternative therapies have proven benefits. Acupuncture, for example, can relieve headaches, muscle aches, and low back pain, she argues. In addition, Ince reports that hypnosis helps injuries heal faster and alleviates fears and phobias. However, Ince maintains that alternative medicine is not for everyone, and she suggests that people consult their doctor before trying unconventional therapies. Ince is a medical writer whose articles have appeared in many national magazines, including *Glamour*, *American Health*, *Redbook*, and *Good Housekeeping*.

As you read, consider the following questions:

1. According to the author, in what areas is acupuncture ineffective?
2. In Ince's opinion, who should not utilize therapeutic massage?
3. List three of the author's suggestions on how to get the best alternative care.

Remember when alternative medicine was the treatment of last resort? Something to turn to only if conventional medicine failed? Fast-forward to the present, when doctors like Judith Peterson, M.D., a professor of physical medicine at Thomas Jefferson University Hospital in Philadelphia, are using acupuncture and herbs as well as surgery, medication, and exercise to help rehabilitate patients from a variety of musculoskeletal injuries. "Alternative therapy is integrated with everything else I do," she says. At the Advocate Medical Group in Park Ridge, Illinois, acupuncturists, chiropractors, homeopaths, nutritionists, massage therapists, and mind-body specialists meet with physicians to plan a team approach to each patient's care. Says medical director Donald W. Novey, M.D., "That way, both patients and doctors know that they can have the benefits of a monitored approach—they can put their toes into cold water and still feel safe."

Ready to take the plunge? This guide will give you an informed insider's perspective. Learn what medical research shows each remedy can—and can't—help; what treatment feels like; how long it should take to see results; when to call it quits; and how to get insurance coverage. Read on—your good health might depend on it!

The Benefits of Acupuncture

Your problem:

Musculoskeletal problems such as sciatica (hip and leg pain), headache, menstrual cramps, tennis elbow, fibromyalgia (stiff, inflamed muscles), muscle pain, osteoarthritis, low back pain, or wrist pain due to carpal tunnel syndrome.

Consider: acupuncture

What research shows:

In 1997, a National Institutes of Health consensus panel found clear evidence of acupuncture's value in relieving muscle pain. [In] November [1999], investigators using magnetic resonance images discovered one way acupuncture works—it calms pain-induced brain activity by 60 to 70 percent.

Acupuncture has also achieved good results in some frustrating medical conditions, including dry mouth caused by the autoimmune condition Sjogren's syndrome, jaw pain caused by temporomandibular joint syndrome, diabetic nerve pain, stroke rehabilitation, asthma, and chronic lung disease. It can also temporarily relieve ringing in the ears, or tinnitus.

What it doesn't help:

Acupuncture is not effective in smoking cessation or promoting weight loss.

What it's like:

At your first visit, the acupuncturist will take a standard medical history, then ask detailed questions about things that may seem far afield (such as your food preferences and when and where you tend to sweat). The physical exam will pay particular attention to your pulse (which is taken in more than one spot) and your tongue, which acupuncturists believe reveals internal changes.

Alternative Medicine Is Gaining Acceptance

Evidence is mounting that conventional medicine does not offer all the answers to preventing illness and curing disease. *World Development Indicators* shows that the U.S. life expectancy rate was only 21st and the U.S. infant mortality rate ranked 27th of other nations studied. The U.S. spends more dollars on health care than other nations and has failed to be one of the leaders in actually providing a healthier quality of life. This fact has opened the door for alternative or complementary medicine (CAM) to be utilized and researched. According to the National Library of Medicine, the terms "complementary medicine" and "alternative medicine" are used interchangeably. In *Mosby's Medical Nursing, & Allied Health Dictionary*, alternative medicine is defined as "any of the systems of medical diagnosis and treatment differing in technique from that of the allopathic practitioner's use of drugs and surgery to treat disease and injury." During 1997, consumers spent between $4 billion and $6 billion on visits to massage therapists, making up approximately 27 percent of the $21.2 billion spent on CAM, and demand continues to increase. In a 1998 *Newsday Magazine* article, it was reported that from 1990 to 1997, there was a 380 percent increase in vitamin usage and a 130 percent increase in the use of herbal supplements. These percentages are staggering. The validity of alternative medicine is increasing throughout the medical industry as consumers experiment and demand options to conventional medicine. This has been a long, hard battle for some of the alternative therapies.

Carrie Bodane and Kenneth Brownson, *Health Care Manager*, March 2002.

For the treatment itself, you'll usually change into a hospital gown and lie down. Sterile needles a hair's width across—often 10 to 20 at a time—will be inserted into selected acupoints.

"Some you won't feel at all; others will have the sting of a mosquito bite," says acupuncturist Lixing Lao, Ph.D., a researcher at the University of Maryland School of Medicine. "The hands and feet are usually more sensitive than the upper arms, thighs, or abdomen. If you are very sensitive, speak up. Your acupuncturist can insert fewer needles."

Typically, the needles are left in place for 20 to 30 minutes. During that time, the points may be stimulated by twirling the needles or applying a small electrical current. Heat may also be used to stimulate the acupuncture points.

After a session you'll most likely feel relaxed; a few people feel energized. If possible, don't go right back to stressful or heavy work right after a session.

It may not be for you if:

• You faint at the sight of needles!

• You are pregnant, bleed easily, or have a pacemaker or breast implants (puncture is a risk). . . .

When to move on:

If there is no improvement after eight sessions, further treatment is unlikely to help.

Benefits of Biofeedback

Your problem:

Muscle tension symptoms (headache, muscle spasm, back pain); migraine headache; circulatory problems due to Raynaud's syndrome; stress, panic, or anxiety disorders; insomnia.

Consider: biofeedback

What research shows:

Biofeedback is an effective treatment for many problems related to muscle tension. It can also be used to train the contraction of specific muscles in order to treat incontinence (it works better than drugs) or to rehabilitate muscle or spinal cord injuries.

Learning how to increase circulation to the fingers or toes can be a very effective treatment for migraine and for Raynaud's syndrome, which have few traditional treatments.

Finally, you can use biofeedback to learn general relaxation for stress management or to treat chronic pain, anxiety, or panic disorders.

What it doesn't help:

Despite claims, there is little solid evidence that it helps attention deficit disorder.

What it's like:

To get the information—the feedback—that will allow you to learn to make changes in body functions, such as blood vessel dilation, body temperature, muscle tension, or heart rate, the practitioner will tape or stick small electrical sensors to your head, hands, and other body parts. You do not have to get undressed.

If the goal is to slow your heart rate (for stress relief, insomnia, or high blood pressure), a pulse monitor will be slipped over your finger. Each time your pulse beats, the sensor will beep and a light will flash.

The therapist will then teach you how breathing more deeply or visualizing a relaxing scene can influence the readings that you see. During a session, you will practice the relaxation technique with constant feedback from the sensors. Between sessions, you will practice the actions on your own, perhaps using a home device. Eventually, you should gain control over your responses and not need the continuous feedback.

It may not be for you if:

• Other treatments (such as meditation, relaxation, or hypnosis) seem to be just as effective for your condition. . . .

When to move on:

• If, after ten sessions, biofeedback fails to relieve your symptoms.

• If your medical problem worsens or if biofeedback therapy that has been helpful suddenly seems to stop working, see your doctor. . . .

Benefits of Hypnosis

Your problem:

Stress-related disorders such as headaches, irritable bowel syndrome, panic attacks, nail biting and hair pulling, and fears and phobias.

Consider: hypnosis

What research shows:

Hypnosis has been shown to reduce pain, whether from a recent injury or chronic problem, and it can also promote healing. [In 1999], Harvard researchers found that when hypnosis was added to standard orthopedic care, patients with a broken foot healed more quickly (as documented by X-ray), walked more easily, and used fewer painkillers.

What it doesn't help:

• Results with smoking cessation aren't encouraging—only about 20 percent of smokers stop—but are just as good as those from other treatments.

What it's like:

You'll spend part of the first visit in discussion with the hypnotist. You need to make sure that you have a good rapport with the practitioner; the hypnotist needs to find out about your specific problem and your learning style in order to help you enter a trance, which is basically a state of heightened awareness and focused concentration.

"Education is a crucial part of the session," says Eric Simon, Ph.D., a psychologist at Tripler Regional Medical Center in Honolulu. "I reassure patients that I have hypnotized more than a thousand people and none of them has ever seen a ghost or been told to bark like a dog. All hypnosis is self-hypnosis, and you are in control."

You will usually be seated in a comfortable chair and told to focus on an object or an image. A trance will be induced by directing your focus to a scene described by the hypnotist. While in a trance state, you are quite susceptible to suggestions given by the therapist to help with your medical problem.

When you are brought back to full awakeness, you may feel as if you have been asleep. Depending on your goal, one or more hypnosis sessions may be needed, and you may be taught how to practice self-hypnosis at home. Roberta Temes, Ph.D., author of *The Complete Idiot's Guide to Hypnosis*, invites her clients to bring a tape recorder so they can re-experience their sessions at home.

It may not be for you if:

• You have symptoms that need a medical workup first.

• You are suicidal or have a personality disorder or psychosis. . . .

When to move on:

Your symptoms have not begun to improve in the time the hypnotist originally estimated.

Benefits of Massage

Your problem:

Muscular symptoms due to back pain, fibromyalgia, carpal tunnel syndrome, tennis elbow, sprains and strains, or stress-related medical conditions (sleep difficulties, digestive disorders, high blood pressure, and headache).

Consider: therapeutic massage

What medical research shows:

Studies have documented massage's ability to increase relaxation, reduce stress, and ease tight and aching muscles.

At the Touch Research Institute of the University of Miami, researchers have shown that massage decreases the stress hormones norepinephrine and cortisol while boosting levels of serotonin (which decline in people who are depressed or in pain), says Maria Hernandez-Reif, Ph.D., director of research. The changes are only temporary but can accumulate with repeated sessions.

Massage also seems to have immunity-boosting effects; according to Hernandez-Reif, studies in breast cancer and HIV have shown that massage therapy increases natural killer cells that fight tumors and viruses.

Specialized lymphatic massage can help reduce certain types of swelling, such as that experienced by some women after breast cancer surgery.

What it doesn't help:

Massage can reduce some symptoms associated with a disease or condition—decreasing fatigue and pain, relieving stress—but it cannot cure it.

What it's like:

Most massages are given while you lie on a padded table. Typically, you remove your clothing and cover yourself with a sheet or large towel. (Some types, such as Shiatsu, are usually done clothed.) The American Massage Therapy Association (AMTA) requires its members to uncover only those parts that are being worked on. To ease friction against the skin, oil or lotion is usually used.

It may not be for you if:

• You have phlebitis (pressure may cause a clot to break away from the swollen vein and lodge in your lung or brain, resulting in a stroke).

• You currently have a rash, infection, or fever. A massage therapist will not work directly over a tumor, a recent incision, an open wound, or swollen or bruised tissues. . . .

When to move on:

If your symptoms worsen or don't improve and you have not noticed other benefits, such as improved sleep or reduced stress.

Benefits of Yoga

Your problem:

Musculoskeletal pain, multiple sclerosis, osteoarthritis, menstrual cramps, asthma, or diabetes.

Consider: yoga

What research shows:

Pain is the primary reason that people start to practice yoga, says Gail Dubinsky, M.D., a yoga instructor and orthopedist in Sebastopol, California.

In one study, patients with osteoarthritis of the hands had less pain and tenderness and were able to move their fingers farther after yoga. In a 1998 study, people with carpal tunnel syndrome lessened their pain through eight weeks of yoga classes, while a control group using traditional wrist splints did not improve.

"Get a diagnosis for your problem, then find a teacher who is experienced in working with that condition," advises Marian Garfinkel of Hahnemann University in Philadelphia, lead researcher for the two studies. Both the Arthritis Foundation and the National Multiple Sclerosis Society recommend yoga.

Yoga can also be beneficial for other conditions. When adult asthmatics took yoga classes for 16 weeks, they were more able to exercise without symptoms and used their inhalers less. Dean Ornish, M.D., founder of the Preventive Medicine Research Institute in Sausalito, CA, considers yoga an important part of his lifestyle program for reversing heart disease. And yoga can be helpful to women with menstrual cramps, asthma, and diabetes.

What it doesn't help:

Yoga may improve symptoms associated with a condition, but it cannot cure it.

What it's like:

Yoga instruction can be individual or in a class. Wear stretchy clothes and plan to go barefoot. Shorts or tights will allow the teacher to see how you are positioning your legs so you can move safely. Don't eat for a couple hours prior to class. Your teacher needs to know about any medical concerns or physical limitations or injuries you may have and should know how to adapt the poses for your body type and level of strength and flexibility.

It may not be for you if:

• You have high blood pressure, heart problems, or serious diabetes; these may preclude doing strenuous types of yoga, such as Ashtanga. . . .

When to move on:

If your symptoms worsen or you haven't noticed other benefits such as improved sleep or reduced stress.

How to Get the Best Care

No matter what treatment you're considering, make sure you:

Get a diagnosis: Alternative care should not be used to treat symptoms without having a clear idea of what is behind them. "Diagnosis is still the most important thing in planning your health care," says Judith Peterson, M.D.

Know your practitioner: Ask about licensure, training, and experience in treating others with your condition. Beware of a practitioner who wants you to cut off standard medical care or refuses to communicate with your other doctors.

Find out how many treatments you'll need: A good practitioner will be able to estimate how many sessions it will take for you to feel better.

Respect your individuality: Not everyone benefits from the same techniques, stresses Donald Novey, M.D. "One thing doesn't work for everybody, and when you think about it, even physicians don't believe that or there wouldn't be 15 different classes of drugs to treat high blood pressure," he says.

Do your part: Most alternative practitioners won't just work on you in their office; they'll want you to make changes in your exercise and diet habits and find ways to reduce your stress.

Will Your Insurance Pay?

Touting coverage for alternative medicine is the hottest trend in insurance marketing. The problem? What you get is less than what you might imagine from the ads and brochures. Four questions to ask before signing up:

1. Is it a discount network or a fully integrated benefit? In many plans, all you get is access to a group of alternative health practitioners who have agreed to give discounts to people with the insurance plan. In other words, the insurer negotiated the deal but isn't paying a penny toward the care.

"The discount may be trivial (only 10 to 15 percent) relative to the extra premium you are paying. You may be better off taking lower-priced insurance and paying for alternative health care yourself," says Kenneth Pelletier, Ph.D., senior research scholar at the Stanford Center for Research on Disease Prevention.

2. Does it include the providers you want? Each plan differs in the types of alternative health care it includes. And if the provider you prefer isn't in a network, it may not be worth the money.

3. How easy is it to get appointments? Some plans let you go directly to a practitioner (often paying a higher percentage of the fee yourself); others require a referral from a primary care physician or a letter explaining why the treatment is medically necessary.

4. What are the limits on benefits? All of the plans limit either the cost or number of visits covered each year, cautions Pelletier. "For example, the brochure may say acupuncture is covered, but the fine print shows a limit of four visits a year. The research on acupuncture shows that there is virtually nothing that can be successfully treated with only four visits," he says. "Or there may be a limit on total alternative care, so you have to pick and choose to avoid getting stuck with large bills."

"*Direct harm may occur to the patient due to use of dangerous, often nonstandardized treatments.*"

Alternative Therapies Are Harmful

Roland J. Lamarine

According to Roland J. Lamarine in the following viewpoint, many people view alternative therapies as harmless options to conventional medicine. However, he argues, alternative medicine is based on unscientific, unproven theories. Lamarine asserts that alternative therapies can actually harm patients by subjecting them to dangerous treatments. Lamarine maintains that people should be skeptical of therapies that are not subjected to the same rigorous tests as are conventional medical treatments. Lamarine is on the faculty of the Department of Health and Community Services at California State University, Chico.

As you read, consider the following questions:
1. How does the author define alternative medicine?
2. According to Lamarine, on what is good science based?
3. What are two harms associated with alternative therapies, as stated by the author?

Roland J. Lamarine, "Alternative Medicine: More than Just a Harmless Option," *Journal of School Health*, vol. 71, March 2001, p. 114. Copyright © 2001 by American School Health Association, Kent, Ohio. Reproduced by permission.

A fourth grade teacher learns that a nine-year-old student in her class has been diagnosed with a brain tumor. After surgery to remove the growth, the child's physicians recommend chemotherapy and radiotherapy. This treatment offers a survival rate greater than 50%. After talking to friends and a "well-informed" clerk at the local health food store, the child's parents learn that sharks do not develop cancer because they are built of cartilage, which contains anti-cancer agents. They confide in the teacher that chemotherapy and radiotherapy are toxic and dangerous interventions, but shark cartilage is organic, pure, and natural. They suggest that using this "home remedy" will provide their child with greater autonomy and self-determination in addressing her illness. They decide to pursue the natural therapy.

This scenario, which still may not represent the norm, becomes more common with each passing year. At the beginning of a new millennium, alternative medical practices continue to emerge and to thrive. During 1990, Americans paid more visits to alternative medical practitioners than to all primary care physicians combined, spending an estimated $13.7 billion on unproven and untested remedies. Between 1990 and 1997, use of alternative medical therapies increased from 34% to 42% of Americans, with a conservative estimate of $21 billion in expenditures in 1997. . . .

Background on Alternative Medicine

Several sources provide useful definitions of alternative medicine. Sometimes called complementary medicine, alternative therapies encompass a range of approaches including everything from dietary supplements, herbs, and biological agents to manual healing, bioelectromagnetics, mind-body interventions, and alternative medical practices. Alternative medicine includes therapies employed as part of traditional medicine and some approaches clearly exposed as quackery. This paper defines alternative medicine as unproven, untested, and disproven approaches. Some forms of conventional medicine also fall within this definition as well. One poignant description of alternative medicine suggests, "There is no alternative medicine. There is only scientifically proven, evidence-based medicine supported by solid data or unproven medicine for which scientific evidence is lacking." Using this criterion, most of alternative medicine and much of conventional medicine, would be abandoned until sufficient testing were completed. New therapies should, where feasible, be tested scientifically for efficacy and safety.

Characteristics of Users of Alternative Medicine

Recent research provides a profile of people most likely to use alternative medicine. Compared to nonusers, alternative medicine users were better educated, more often reported lower than average health status, and were more likely to view alternative health care as more congruent with their own values, beliefs, and philosophies toward health and life.

The main benefit reported by users of alternative medicine was relief from symptoms of their illness. Surprisingly, users were not significantly more likely to report dissatisfaction or distrust of conventional medicine except for approximately 5% who relied primarily on alternative care to the exclusion of conventional medicine.

Evidence suggests that somatization characterizes many current users of alternative medicine. Somatizers seem more finely attuned to their bodies' aches and pains, more likely to attribute physical discomfort to disease, and more likely to seek medical assistance for what often appear to be illnesses of psychosomatic origin.

A recent study that surveyed women who received standard therapy for early-stage breast cancer indicated that, within this group, users of alternative medicine reported more depression, greater fear of recurrence, and less robust mental health. Those patients who had not used alternative medicine prior to their cancer, but began to use alternative therapies after their diagnosis, presented more evidence of psychological fragility including lower levels of sexual satisfaction, greater fear of recurrence, and more severe physical symptoms. Similar findings were noted in a study of patients with brain tumors.

Characteristics of Alternative Medicine

Alternative therapies are often described as natural, organic, holistic, or a combination of all three. The term "holistic" is often associated with anything good and wholesome, which integrates physical, mental, emotional, and spiritual dimensions into a natural, vital, life-affirming unity. Unlike the reductionistic, scientific approach of evidence-based medical regimens, much of alternative medicine by contrast adopts an expansionist, all-inclusive approach. Some alternative therapies are characterized by attempts to address the needs of the whole person in a spiritual belief system that requires not only faith in the practitioner and in the practice, but foremost, faith in oneself as the ultimate healer in the self-care system.

Alternative vs. Conventional Medicine

In recent years, much of conventional medicine has adopted the scientific and reductionistic philosophy of René Descartes, while alternative therapies continue to regularly cross the line into the mystical domain offering an appealing blend of pseudoscience and spirituality. Clearly many Americans prefer an optimistic therapy that offers both medicine for the body and nourishment for the soul. Scientifically based medicine subscribes to a more rigorous, evidence-based, self-critical methodology that is realistic and probabilistic, and may be less likely to offer falsely optimistic prognoses. Sometimes this approach may be distasteful, hurtful, and unpleasant to patients.

Since early research indicated the placebo effect may account for fully one-third of medically assisted recoveries, an argument can be made supporting falsely optimistic prognoses that may act as mental placebos for patients. In some instances conventional medicine may be at a disadvantage in competition with alternative therapies in terms of allaying fears. Scientific reality constrains conventional medicine. Truth and honesty do not permit ethically the encouragement of false hope and questionable therapeutic pursuits.

The apparent successes attributed to unproven and discredited therapies can be explained by a variety of possibilities. The previously mentioned placebo effect has been shown to sometimes provide symptom relief, if not actual cures. Variability in symptoms from person-to-person and time-to-time can account for apparent improvement in health status following use of alternative therapies, as well as conventional therapies. Time-related effects can provide misleading and misperceived outcomes. A delay of impact may occur from a conventional treatment that patients mistakenly attribute to the more recent alternative therapy, when the earlier conventional treatment was in fact the causal agent.

Alternative Therapies Should Be Scientifically Tested

It is time for the scientific community to stop giving alternative medicine a free ride. There cannot be two kinds of medicine—conventional and alternative. There is only medicine that has been adequately tested and medicine that has not, medicine that works and medicine that may or may not work. Once a treatment has been tested rigorously, it no longer matters whether it was considered alternative at the outset. If it is found to be reasonably safe and effective, it will be accepted. But assertions, speculation, and testimonials do not substitute for evidence. Alternative treatments should be subjected to scientific testing no less rigorous than that required for conventional treatments.

Marcia Angell and Jerome P. Kassirer, *Skeptical Inquirer*, January/February 1999.

Patients commonly blend alternative and conventional therapies, then attribute beneficial outcomes to the wrong therapy. Reporting bias is a major contributor to the undeserved reputation for some worthless therapies. Even some "documented" remissions can occur by chance. It is necessary to know the denominators in fractions. How many patients were "cured" out of how many treated? Probability theory tells us that one in 20 cases prove "significant" due to chance alone.

When conventional therapies emerge from trials employing scientific methods, they have been developed using testable methodologies. Results are honestly and openly published in peer-reviewed journals which invite, even encourage, critical analysis and debate. Objective methodologies are utilized and results must be repeatable by different and independent researchers, using objective, standardized methodologies such as randomized, controlled trials.

Some alternative treatments attain success in good measure by offering hope to the hopeless. In cases of serious illness, where conventional medicine is unable to honestly offer cure, patients may become desperate for survival and hope. Whereas the evidence-based, conventional practitioner's explanations can be complex, sometimes those who subscribe to alternative therapies, unrestrained by sound science, can offer simplistic, optimistic solutions.

Science or Pseudoscience?

Science entails more than a compilation of facts, principles, and laws. Science provides a way of examining the world and making sense of it. The scientific method, when understood, provides perhaps the most powerful and awe-inspiring idea developed by humans. Science, when conducted properly, protects us from ourselves. It protects us from common sense which, though desirable, still limits us to the familiar. Science provides a mechanism for circumventing traditions that can be stifling. Most importantly, for primates attracted to dominance hierarchies, science protects us against arguments from authority. Good science is based on causality and probability. Causality may be viewed as the idea that present actions lead to future outcomes, while probability suggests that outcomes occur more often when causes are present than when they are absent, but that they do not always follow causes.

Use of standard scientific methodology protects against a virtual plethora of human errors including inaccurate observation, overgeneralization, selective observation, rationalization, illogical reasoning, ego-involvement in understanding, premature closure of inquiry, and mystification. Scientific knowledge is precise and repeatable, and science "demands adequate reason, coherent argument, rigorous standards of evidence and honesty . . . it is a way to call the bluff of those who may only pretend to knowledge . . . a bulwark against mysticism, against superstition, against religion misapplied," [as stated by Carl Sagan in *The Demon-Haunted World*.]

Pseudoscience rationalizes its failures with explanations that do not lend themselves to critical evaluation. Failures may be underreported by pseudoscientific practitioners, or reasons for failures may be directed back at the victim, because within the context of holistic medicine, therapeutic failure can reflect a failure on the part of the patient to believe deeply enough in the therapy or to eliminate negative thought. Keep in mind that the practice of pseudoscience is not restricted only to practitioners of alternative medicine.

Harm Associated with Use of Alternative Therapy

One often encounters rationalizations such as "What's the harm of using alternative therapy? Who knows, maybe it will help?" This sort of simplistic thinking overlooks several significant dangers associated with the use of alternative medicine, defined as unproven, untested, or disproven therapies.

First, such therapies can result in economic harm to the user, who might expend valuable economic resources on questionable protocols, resources that could be better spent on proven remedies.

Second, direct harm may occur to the patient due to use of dangerous, often nonstandardized treatments. Reports of cyanide toxicity from laetrile and ruptured colons associated with coffee enemas are examples of such dangers.

Third, indirect harm may result from failure to receive helpful therapies or from delays in accepting conventional treatments that may be more effective at an earlier stage of the disease.

Fourth, social harm may derive from individual role modeling of undesirable behaviors. Perhaps a beloved relative selects an alternative therapy, which then increases its validity in the eyes of younger family members. Organized groups advocating for alternative therapies can breed distrust of established institutions, thereby interfering with their ability to provide beneficial services.

The vignette presented at the beginning of this paper, describing a nine-year-old girl with a brain tumor whose parents opted for shark cartilage in lieu of conventional therapy, was based on an actual experience at Alberta Children's Hospital in Calgary, Alberta, Canada. The child in question subsequently died, bringing home in chillingly clear detail, one tragic consequence associated with use of unproven therapies. . . .

Preparing Tomorrow's Adults

The apparent increase in the number of adult Americans who uncritically accept alternative therapies, or for that matter conventional therapies, without demanding to know the scientific evidence supporting their efficacy may indicate a failure to properly educate the public in a fundamental understanding of the scientific method and its application to the health field. This situation may also indicate a need for more and better consumer health education which could prepare tomorrow's adults to become more discerning and objective judges of the efficacy of the medical products and practices available to them.

> *"Homeopathy has been used for 200 years, and its safety and efficacy have stood the test of time."*

Homeopathic Remedies Are Effective

Eric L. Foxman

In the following viewpoint Eric L. Foxman argues that homeopathy—a therapy that administers minute doses of a substance that, in a healthy person, would produce symptoms similar to the illness—is a safe and effective therapy. He maintains that, like vaccines, homeopathic medicines enhance the body's healing process by stimulating the immune system. By administering small doses of medicine, homeopathy avoids the side effects associated with conventional drug treatments, according to Foxman. Foxman is a pharmacist and consultant to complementary pharmaceutical manufacturers.

As you read, consider the following questions:
1. What did Samuel Hahnemann name his approach to medicine?
2. What are the two goals of combination remedies, as reported by Foxman?
3. Name three famous supporters of homeopathy listed by the author.

Eric L. Foxman, "Homeopathy," *Better Nutrition*, vol. 61, December 1999, p. 44. Copyright © 1999 by Primedia Intertec. Reproduced by permission.

After decades of relative obscurity, homeopathy is making a phenomenal comeback. How has this happened? How will this help you, the consumer of natural medical therapies, regain and maintain your health?

Today's educated consumer is confronted with many choices. Some are new and not well proven. Others promise what seems to be impossible. Repeatedly, side effects of new medicines become apparent over time, or their effectiveness doesn't live up to the initial hype. However, homeopathy has been used for 200 years, and its safety and efficacy have stood the test of time.

What Is Homeopathy?

Homeopathy owes its origin to a man with a unique set of talents—Samuel Hahnemann. This physician, medical school lecturer, chemist, and translator was well versed in the medical texts of five languages. While pursuing his written work, he began to research the use of quinine (a substance purified from the bark of the cinchona tree) on malaria. Hahnemann tested the effect of quinine and other substances on healthy subjects; through careful observation, he recorded these effects as "symptom pictures," or "provings."

Hahnemann then conducted very thorough exams with his patients, going beyond the physical symptoms of the illness. He was keenly interested in changes in the patient's general health, their feelings and mental outlook, and how their symptoms varied with different circumstances (e.g., at night, when exposed to warm air, with foods). Hahnemann matched the patient's symptoms to the "symptom pictures" of the substances he had researched. He then administered a diluted preparation of the matching compound.

The Healing Process

Hahnemann realized symptoms are an expression of the healing process. By using the diluted matching preparations, the innate healing steps are stimulated to begin or continue their natural course. Hahnemann named this approach: "Similia similibus curantur" or "Likes are cured by likes," also called the Law of Similars. In other words, homeopathic therapy uses a medicinal substance with a "symptom picture" that is most similar to the symptoms of the person who is sick. Thus, homeopathy works with the body's inherent recovery process.

At first glance, the use of a "similar" substance may seem confusing, or even unreasonable. But there are numerous examples in everyday medicine of this phenomenon. Vaccination is a related process which is designed to elicit the body's natural healing process by, in a sense, "fooling" the body into thinking that an attenuated form of a virus is the genuine article, for example.

From his extensive medical experience, Hahnemann realized even small amounts of strong substances can have deleterious effects. Consequently, he developed a serial dilution method and special mixing method; this results in the safest cure without aggravating or worsening the symptoms. It has been said that this method is an energetic process, which releases the therapeutic properties of the substance into the mixture. Through this, homeopathy takes advantage of the curative character of each remedy, and, at the same time, eliminates concern regarding undesirable side effects.

In addition to the use of homeopathically prepared substances, the homeopathic practitioner works with all factors which can influence a patient's well being, including: good diet, hygiene, exercise, coping with family, work, spirituality, and stress, as well as environmental factors. Hahnemann's approach was a true forerunner of that of today's holistic physician.

How Do I Use Homeopathic Products?

Single remedies. There are two types of homeopathic products. First are the homeopathic "single" remedies. To use these properly, consumers must know the fine subtleties of homeopathic practice. There are intricacies in the choice of the proper remedy for which study and careful consideration are required. For instance, in the case of a cough—Is it deep and rasping with lots of phlegm and made worse when drinking cold fluids? Or is it a dry tickling cough that occurs every few minutes and seems better in the evening? Different remedies are appropriate for each, and the choice may be further influenced by other factors about the individual patient. For both practitioners and consumers familiar with this level of detail, single homeopathic remedies can be a perfect match. Some of these single remedies are also powerful tools for serious conditions when used by a trained homeopathic practitioner.

Healing a Cold

Homeopathy is a system that attempts to stimulate the body to heal itself. I realized that all symptoms, no matter how uncomfortable they are, represent the body's attempt to restore itself to health. So instead of trying to dry up the runny nose from a cold with antihistamines, a homeopath will use a remedy that will stimulate the body to move in the direction it is already going, and, in the process, clear the runny nose!

It is a system that looks at individuals and not at diseases. Each of us suffers a cold in his or her unique way. Yet conventional medicine makes the assumption that all colds are alike and offers a common series of drugs, something to dry the nose, something to bring down the fever, something to suppress the cough, something to ease the headache. Homeopathy, on the other hand, looks for the one substance that will cure the *individual* case. The person with a beginning cold, characterized by slow onset, aching, loss of appetite, chills, and a desire to be left alone will need a different remedy than the person whose cold comes on a bit quicker and is characterized by intense sneezing, a runny nose that burns the upper lip, a desire for hot drinks, a bone chilling coldness, and a desire *not* to be left alone. We characterize both as *colds*, but they are expressed differently, and, therefore, are in need of different homeopathic remedies.

Julian Winston, National Center for Homeopathy, 2002.

Combination remedies. On the other hand, most manufacturers also sell combination products for everyday ailments, such as allergies, headache, and cold and flu symptoms. These combinations are formulated to affect a wide range of symptoms commonly experienced by a large percentage of the population. By using more than one component, the formulation can accomplish two goals:

1) Different ingredients can be present to help with the varying subtleties of the symptoms (for example, the different types of coughs); this is particularly helpful when the

character of the illness changes during the course of the health-restoring process.

2) More than one avenue can be used to help the recovery process of related symptoms. For example, a cold-and-flu remedy can contain an ingredient for fever, another ingredient for nasal congestion, and a third for the sore throat which accompanies the flu symptoms. When formulated in this manner, a combination product can be easy for the consumer to use, especially those new to this form of complementary medicine.

A Safe Alternative

With a clearly labeled indication and easy directions for use, homeopathic products provide a simple and effective choice for your natural health care needs. With the knowledge that homeopathy has been used safely for decades, you have an attractive and safe alternative to more costly, and potentially troublesome, conventional drugs. As with any responsible therapeutic modality, some medical circumstances—acute trauma and life-threatening conditions—are best treated by a trained medical practitioner. A proper medical diagnosis is necessary for those serious, life-threatening conditions. In these situations, it would be irresponsible for patients to attempt to treat themselves with any type of medicine, whether complementary or conventional. However, most common everyday health problems can be appropriately, adequately, and safely treated using homeopathic medicines available at your health food store.

Homeopathy's Long History of Use in the United States

After Hahnemann's initial successes in Germany, homeopathy was brought to [the United States] in the early 1830s. Its phenomenal success in the 19th century was due to extensive use by 9 to 14 percent of all medical doctors. This success led to an unfortunate backlash by "regular" doctors, the then-fledgling American Medical Association, a couple of non-homeopathic pharmaceutical companies, a few non-homeopathic pharmacies, and a collection of non-homeopathic/non-Eclectic medical associations, all of which attempted to suppress homeopathy and Eclectic [holistic, "nature"] Medicine. The advent of sulfa drugs and antibiotics in the first half of this century continued to limit the number of physicians who used homeopathic medicines.

Yet, with over 150 years of experience, and millions of patients treated, there have been no reports of adverse effects with homeopathy. No homeopathic medicine has been recalled for medically-related problems.

Are Homeopathic Medicines Used Elsewhere?

The World Health Organization reports that homeopathy is the second-most-widely-used medical modality for primary health care around the world. In Europe, the medical acceptance of homeopathy is very high, including its use by 70 to 80 percent of German physicians and one third of French doctors. The majority of pharmacies in Europe stock homeopathic medicines. The top-selling cold and flu remedy and the number-one-selling motion-sickness product in Europe are both homeopathic. And, insurance plans in most European countries cover homeopathic medicines. While other countries may seem to have a head start on homeopathy, the growth in the United States is now dramatic. A study from 1993 revealed 2 and one-half million Americans were using homeopathic products. In the interim, the market has continued to grow at a rate of 15 to 20 percent annually, with the latest estimates at $270 million per year.

How Are Homeopathic Products Regulated?

Homeopathy remedies have a unique status. They must also meet the exacting requirements of the *Homeopathic Pharmacopoeia of the United States* (HPUS). Federal law and the Food and Drug Administration (FDA) identify this book as the only official standard for homeopathic manufacturing and quality. No other complementary therapy has such a resource document.

As the decade comes to a close, the homeopathic movement is rapidly regaining favor, both among doctors and patients. Increasingly, the original ideas of Hahnemann—to work with the inherent curative powers of the human body—are again being discovered as universal truths which can be vigorously applied and utilized to help patients in a variety of medical situations.

Requirements for homeopathic drugs:
- registration of the company with the FDA
- Federal and state inspections of manufacturing facilities
- review of formulas and labeling by FDA
- Federal labeling requirements
- quality-control testing and documentation
- stability monitoring
- good manufacturing practices—both FDA and HPUS
- extensive documentation of manufacturing steps
- label and inventory control
- recall and complaint resolution procedures
- Federal "Adverse Event" tracking system

Who Uses Homeopathy?

Prominent Americans in many fields have been ardent users and supporters of homeopathy, including Daniel Webster, Louisa May Alcott, Samuel Morse, Henry Longfellow, Horace Greeley, Harriet Beecher Stowe, Nathaniel Hawthorne, John Rockefeller, and three U.S. Presidents: Chester A. Arthur, James Garfield, and William McKinley. More recent examples include actress Jane Seymour, the British Royal Family, and violin virtuoso, Yehudi Menuhin.

It is difficult to design and implement conventional, double-blind clinical trials for homeopathy. Homeopathic therapy is based on the uniqueness of each patient; each person's illness is treated individually, and not as part of a statistical mass. For this reason, homeopathy is sometimes ignored by the conventional medical establishment. A more appropriate point of view is to acknowledge that homeopathy does not easily fit this conventional mold, but, rather, is better judged on the obvious evidence of its accumulated success, which is built one patient at a time. The recent turn toward "evidence-based" medicine is a step in this direction.

Nevertheless, a . . . 1999 study which appeared in *Inflammation Research*, by P. Belon, and colleagues ("Inhibition of human basophil degranulation by successive histamine dilutions: results of a European multi-centre trial"), proved—once and for all—that the effects of homeopathic dilutions can, indeed, be measured using mainstream, conventional-medicine, empirical parameters.

| *"There is no evidence that homeopathy is any more effective than placebo therapy."*

Homeopathic Remedies Are Ineffective

Stephen Barrett

According to Stephen Barrett in the following viewpoint, homeopathy is a quack therapy that is based on superstition instead of science. Homeopathic remedies consist of extremely diluted substances that are intended to stimulate the body's natural immune system. Barrett argues that these substances are diluted to the point that no molecules of the active ingredient remain. Thus, he contends, any relief experienced by patients using homeopathic remedies is due to the placebo effect, not the actual medicine. Stephen Barrett, a retired psychiatrist, has achieved national renown as an author, editor, and consumer advocate.

As you read, consider the following questions:

1. Why, according to Barrett, did eighteenth century medical practitioners begin using homeopathic remedies?
2. In Barrett's opinion, how do homeopathic treatments differ from vaccines?
3. Why is it impossible to validate the ingredients of homeopathic medicines, as reported by the author?

Homeopathic "remedies" enjoy a unique status in the health marketplace: They are the only category of quack products legally marketable as drugs. This situation is the result of two circumstances. First, the 1938 Federal Food, Drug, and Cosmetic Act, which was shepherded through Congress by a homeopathic physician who was a senator, recognizes as drugs all substances included in the *Homeopathic Pharmacopeia of the United States.* Second, the FDA [Food and Drug Administration] has not held homeopathic products to the same standards as other drugs. Today they are marketed in health-food stores, in pharmacies, in practitioner offices, by multilevel distributors, through the mail, and on the Internet.

Basic Misbeliefs

Samuel Hahnemann (1755–1843), a German physician, began formulating homeopathy's basic principles in the late 1700s. Hahnemann was justifiably distressed about bloodletting, leeching, purging, and other medical procedures of his day that did far more harm than good. Thinking that these treatments were intended to "balance the body's 'humors' by opposite effects," he developed his "law of similars"—a notion that symptoms of disease can be cured by extremely small amounts of substances that produce similar symptoms in healthy people when administered in large amounts. The word "homeopathy" is derived from the Greek words *homoios* (similar) and *pathos* (suffering or disease).

Hahnemann and his early followers conducted "provings" in which they administered herbs, minerals, and other substances to healthy people, including themselves, and kept detailed records of what they observed. Later these records were compiled into lengthy reference books called *materia medica*, which are used to match a patient's symptoms with a "corresponding" drug.

Hahnemann declared that diseases represent a disturbance in the body's ability to heal itself and that only a small stimulus is needed to begin the healing process. He also claimed that chronic diseases were manifestations of a suppressed itch (*psora*), a kind of miasma or evil spirit. At first he used small doses of accepted medications. But later he used enormous dilutions and theorized that the smaller the dose, the more powerful the effect—a notion commonly referred to as the "law of infinitesimals." That, of course, is just the opposite of the dose-response relationship that pharmacologists have demonstrated.

No Scientific Testing

The basis for inclusion in the *Homeopathic Pharmacopeia* is not modern scientific testing, but homeopathic "provings" conducted during the 1800s and early 1900s. The current (ninth) edition describes how more than a thousand substances are prepared for homeopathic use. It does not identify the symptoms or diseases for which homeopathic products should be used; that is decided by the practitioner (or manufacturer). The fact that substances listed in the *Homeopathic Pharmacopeia* are legally recognized as "drugs" does not mean that either the law or the FDA recognizes them as effective.

Because homeopathic remedies were actually less dangerous than those of nineteenth-century medical orthodoxy, many medical practitioners began using them. At the turn of the twentieth century, homeopathy had about 14,000 practitioners and 22 schools in the United States. But as medical science and medical education advanced, homeopathy declined sharply in America, where its schools either closed or converted to modern methods. The last pure homeopathic school in this country closed during the 1920s.

Many homeopaths maintain that certain people have a special affinity to a particular remedy (their "constitutional remedy") and will respond to it for a variety of ailments. Such remedies can be prescribed according to the person's "constitutional type"—named after the corresponding remedy in a manner resembling astrologic typing. The "Ignatia Type," for example, is said to be nervous and often tearful, and to dislike tobacco smoke. The typical "Pulsatilla" is a young woman, with blond or light-brown hair, blue eyes, and a delicate complexion, who is gentle, fearful, romantic, emotional, and friendly but shy. The "Nux Vomica Type" is said to be aggressive, bellicose, ambitious, and hyperactive. The "Sulfur Type" likes to be independent. And so on. Does this sound to you like a rational basis for diagnosis and treatment?

The "Remedies" Are Placebos

Homeopathic products are made from minerals, botanical substances, and several other sources. If the original substance is soluble, one part is diluted with either nine or ninety-nine parts of distilled water and/or alcohol and shaken vigorously (succussed); if insoluble, it is finely ground and pulverized in similar proportions with powdered lactose (milk sugar). One part of the diluted medicine is then further diluted, and the process is repeated until the desired concentration is reached. Dilutions of 1 to 10 are designated by the Roman numeral X (1X = 1/10, 3X = 1/1,000, 6X = 1/1,000,000). Similarly, dilutions of 1 to 100 are designated by the Roman numeral C (1C = 1/100, 3C = 1/1,000,000, and so on). Most remedies today range from 6X to 30X, but products of 30C or more are marketed.

A 30X dilution means that the original substance has been diluted 1,000,000,000,000,000,000,000,000,000,000 times. Assuming that a cubic centimeter of water contains 15 drops, this number is greater than the number of drops of water that would fill a container more than 50 times the size of the Earth. Imagine placing a drop of red dye into such a container so that it disperses evenly. Homeopathy's "law of infinitesimals" is the equivalent of saying that any drop of water subsequently removed from that container will possess an essence of redness. Robert L. Park, Ph.D., a prominent physicist who is executive director of The American Physical Society, has noted that since the least amount of a substance in a solution is one molecule, a 30C solution would have to have at least one molecule of the original substance dissolved in a minimum of 1,000,000,000,000,000,000,000,000,000,000,000,000,000,000,000,000,000,000,000,000,000,000 molecules of water. This would require a container more than 30,000,000,000 times the size of the Earth.

Oscillococcinum, a 200C product "for the relief of colds and flu-like symptoms," involves "dilutions" that are even more far-fetched. Its "active ingredient" is prepared by incubating small amounts of a freshly killed duck's liver and heart for 40 days. The resultant solution is then filtered, freeze-dried, rehydrated, repeatedly diluted, and impregnated into sugar granules. If a single molecule of the duck's heart or liver were to survive the dilution, its concentration would be 1 in 100^{200}. This huge number, which has 400 zeroes, is vastly greater than the estimated number of molecules in the universe (about one googol, which is a 1 followed by 100 zeroes). In its February 17, 1997, issue, *U.S. News & World Report* noted that only one duck per year is needed to manufacture the product, which had total sales of $20 million in 1996. The magazine dubbed that unlucky bird "the $20-million duck."

Lack of Positive Findings

Several rigorous trials of homeopathy in human medicine have been performed in recent years. According to these randomized, placebo-controlled, double-blind trials, homeopathic "remedies" are not effective:

- in the treatment of adenoid vegetations (abnormal glandular growths) in children,
- for controlling pain and infection after a total abdominal hysterectomy, and
- for preventing migraines.

Furthermore, none of the studies that have generated positive findings has been replicated with such findings, the methodological quality of these studies has been questionable, and the better studies of homeopathy have tended not to generate positive findings.

David W. Ramey, *Priorities for Health*, November 1, 2000.

Actually, the laws of chemistry state that there is a limit to the dilution that can be made without losing the original substance altogether. This limit, which is related to Avogadro's number, corresponds to homeopathic potencies of 12C or 24X (1 part in 10^{24}). Hahnemann himself realized that there is virtually no chance that even one molecule of original substance would remain after extreme dilutions. But he believed that the vigorous shaking or pulverizing with each step of dilution leaves behind a "spirit-like" essence—"no longer perceptible to the senses"—which cures by reviving the body's "vital force." Modern proponents assert that even when the last molecule is gone, a "memory" of the substance is retained. This notion is unsubstantiated. Moreover, if it were true, every substance encountered by a molecule of water might imprint an "essence" that could exert powerful (and unpredictable) medicinal effects when ingested by a person.

Many proponents claim that homeopathic products resemble vaccines because both provide a small stimulus that triggers an immune response. This comparison is not valid. The amounts of active ingredients in vaccines are much greater and can be measured. Moreover, immunizations produce antibodies whose concentration in the blood can be measured, but high-dilution homeopathic products produce no measurable response. In addition, vaccines are used preventively, not for curing symptoms. . . .

Unimpressive "Research"

Since many homeopathic remedies contain no detectable amount of active ingredient, it is impossible to test whether they contain what their label says. Unlike most potent drugs, they have not been proven effective against disease by double-blind clinical testing. In fact, the vast majority of homeopathic products have never even been tested.

In 1990, an article in *Review of Epidemiology* analyzed 40 randomized trials that had compared homeopathic treatment with standard treatment, a placebo, or no treatment. The authors concluded that all but three of the trials had major flaws in their design and that only one of those three had reported a positive result. The authors concluded that there is no evidence that homeopathic treatment has any more value than a placebo.

In 1994, the journal *Pediatrics* published an article claiming that homeopathic treatment had been demonstrated to be effective against mild cases of diarrhea among Nicaraguan children. The claim was based on findings that, on certain days, the "treated" group had fewer loose stools than the placebo group. However [researchers W.] Sampson and [W.] London noted: (1) the study used an unreliable and unproved diagnostic and therapeutic scheme, (2) there was no safeguard against product adulteration, (3) treatment selection was arbitrary, (4) the data were oddly grouped and contained errors and inconsistencies, (5) the results had questionable clinical significance, and (6) there was no public health significance because the only remedy needed for mild childhood diarrhea is adequate fluid intake to prevent or correct dehydration.

In 1995, *Prescribe International*, a French journal that evaluates pharmaceutical products, published a literature review that concluded:

> As homeopathic treatments are generally used in conditions with variable outcome or showing spontaneous recovery (hence their placebo-responsiveness), these treatments are widely considered to have an effect in some patients. However, despite the large number of comparative trials carried out to date there is no evidence that homeopathy is any more effective than placebo therapy given in identical conditions.

In December 1996, a lengthy report was published by the Homoeopathic Medicine Research Group (HMRG), an expert panel convened by the Commission of the European Communities. The HMRG included homeopathic physician-researchers and experts in clinical research, clinical pharmacology, biostatistics, and clinical epidemiology. Its aim was to evaluate published and unpublished reports of controlled trials of homeopathic treatment. After examining 184 reports, the panelists concluded: (1) only 17 were designed and reported well enough to be worth considering; (2) in some of these trials, homeopathic approaches may have exerted a greater effect than a placebo or no treatment; and (3) the number of participants in these 17 trials was too small to draw any conclusions about the effectiveness of homeopathic treatment for any specific condition. Simply put: Most homeopathic research is worthless, and no homeopathic product has been proven effective for any therapeutic purpose. The National Council Against Health Fraud has warned that "the sectarian nature of homeopathy raises serious questions about the trustworthiness of homeopathic researchers.". . .

Greater Regulation Is Needed

As far as I can tell, the FDA has never recognized any homeopathic remedy as safe and effective for any medical purpose. In 1995, I filed a Freedom of Information Act request that stated:

> I am interested in learning whether the FDA has: (1) received evidence that any homeopathic remedy, now marketed in this country, is effective against any disease or health problem;

(2) concluded that any homeopathic product now marketed in the United States is effective against any health problem or condition; (3) concluded that homeopathic remedies are generally effective; or (4) concluded that homeopathic remedies are generally not effective. Please send me copies of all documents in your possession that pertain to these questions.

An official from the FDA Center for Drug Evaluation and Research replied that several dozen homeopathic products were approved many years ago, but these approvals were withdrawn by 1970. In other words, after 1970, no homeopathic remedy had FDA [approval] as "safe and effective" for its intended purpose. As far as I can tell, that statement is still true today.

If the FDA required homeopathic remedies to be proven effective in order to remain marketable—the standard it applies to other categories of drugs—homeopathy would face extinction in the United States. However, there is no indication that the agency is considering this. FDA officials regard homeopathy as relatively benign (compared, for example, to unsubstantiated products marketed for cancer and AIDS) and believe that other problems should get enforcement priority. If the FDA attacks homeopathy too vigorously, its proponents might even persuade a lobby-susceptible Congress to rescue them. Regardless of this risk, the FDA should not permit worthless products to be marketed with claims that they are effective.

In 1994, forty-two prominent critics of quackery and pseudoscience asked the agency to curb the sale of homeopathic products. The petition urges the FDA to initiate a rulemaking procedure to require that all over-the-counter (OTC) homeopathic drugs meet the same standards of safety and effectiveness as nonhomeopathic OTC drugs. It also asks for a public warning that although the FDA has permitted homeopathic remedies to be sold, it does not recognize them as effective. The FDA has not yet responded to the petition. However, on March 3, 1998, at a symposium sponsored by *Good Housekeeping* magazine, former FDA Commissioner David A. Kessler, M.D., J.D., acknowledged that homeopathic remedies do not work but that he did not attempt to ban them because he felt that Congress would not support a ban.

"The world of herbal medicine offers a wide range of applications and treatments."

Herbal Supplements Are Beneficial

Anne McIntyre

Anne McIntyre argues in the following viewpoint that herbal supplements can relieve a variety of physical and mental ailments. Ginkgo, for example, has been used for centuries to enhance memory and improve brain function, she contends. According to McIntyre, many other herbs are available that fight disease and retard the aging process. She recommends that people with chronic or serious health issues consult an herbalist before taking herbal supplements. McIntyre is a medical herbalist and the former director of the National Institute of Medical Herbalists.

As you read, consider the following questions:

1. According to the author, what are the health benefits of echinacea?
2. For what is ginger a remedy, as reported by McIntyre?
3. As stated by the author, what is St. John's wort used to treat?

Herbs, those "old fashioned" medicines, the stuff of "old wives tales" are being rightfully reinstated at the forefront of modern medicine. Certainly the wealth of articles that appear daily in the press would confirm that their age-old value is being increasingly recognised and that recent research not only validates their ancient medicinal uses but also takes this a few steps further by helping us to understand the biochemical mechanisms involved. Take ginkgo for example, the tree that could be as old as 200 million years, known as the living fossil, the Memory Tree, the Tree of Knowledge and the Plant of Youth, used in Chinese medicine for 5000 years. Apparently today 2000 tons of ginkgo leaf are being harvested a year worldwide and made into a variety of preparations to protect the heart and circulation from the ravages of the ageing process. It is being recommended for improving memory, tinnitus, Raynaud's disease, helping to prevent heart attack, stroke and Alzheimer's disease. Studies have repeatedly shown that elderly people whose mental capacity has deteriorated and who are becoming absent-minded and forgetful have seen some improvement using ginkgo through its significant effect upon cerebral circulation.

Substantial sums of money are being poured into research into the world of plant medicines as scientists continue to search for remedies for devastating illness such as heart disease and cancer. Recently we have heard how a substance derived from the bark of an African willow tree could revolutionise the treatment of cancer by initiating a new way to stop tumour growth. Extracts from the bark of the African Bush Willow (*Combretum caffrum*) have been shown to shut down blood vessels supplying oxygen and nutrients to tumours, thereby inhibiting their growth. Similarly, research has shown that numerous other herbs look hopeful for cancer treatment, including the American yew tree, the Madagascan periwinkle, borage and a Chinese herb called campotheca.

A Variety of Uses

The world of herbal medicine offers a wide range of applications and treatments on several different levels, ranging from everyday over-the-counter remedies for more symptomatic relief of minor ailments, to individualised prescriptions prepared specifically for patients after in depth consultation with a qualified medical herbalist. Certainly herbs have their place as self-help for minor infections, coughs, colds, catarrh, stomach upsets, indigestion, constipation and so on. The wealth of information that abounds today about herbs is enabling people to make increasingly informed decisions about the specific remedies they choose to self-administer. Take Echinacea for example, currently the most popular American herbal remedy, available not only from herbal suppliers and health food shops but also the high street chemists. An excellent remedy for almost all minor infections that really works, available generally in tincture form. The sooner taken, i.e. at first signs of infection, the better, and best taken in doses of ¼–½ tsp. every 2 hours for maximum effect. Purple coneflower (*Echinacea purpurea/angustifolia*) has an antibiotic and antifungal effect, an interferon-like antiviral action and an anti-allergenic effect. This means it can be taken at the first signs of sore throats, colds, chest infections, tonsillitis, glandular fever for example, as well as for more chronic problems such as candida and post-viral syndrome. Taken in hot water it stimulates the circulation and promotes sweating, helping to bring down fevers. As a blood cleanser Echinacea helps clear the skin of infections and to relieve allergies such as urticaria and eczema. It is a great remedy for people whose deficient immune system makes them prone to one infection after another.

Ginger is another wonderful remedy for treating infections and enhancing immunity and ideal for home use. Hot ginger root tea tastes delicious and can be taken at the onset of a sore throat, cold or flu, when feeling tired, chilly or achy, to promote perspiration, bring down a fever and clear catarrh. Its pungency and warming properties have a stimulating effect on the heart and circulation, creating a feeling of warmth and well-being. It invigorates the digestion and moves stagnation of food and subsequent accumulation of toxins, which has a far-reaching effect throughout the body, increasing general health and vitality and enhancing immunity. Ginger makes an excellent remedy for nausea, stomach and bowel infections, wind and colic. Recent research has shown that ginger inhibits clotting and thins the blood, it lowers harmful blood cholesterol and reduces blood pressure. Similar warming remedies that make delicious "cocktails" in hot decoctions with ginger include cinnamon, cloves (avoid during pregnancy) and cardamom. Taken on a regular basis they increase energy, lift the spirits, keep you warm in the winter and help prevent seasonal affective disorder (SAD).

The Herbal Prozac

Another well researched herb that grows daily in popularity is St John's wort (*Hypericum perforatum*), a marvellous remedy for the nervous system, relaxing tension and anxiety and lifting the spirits. Research confirms its ancient use as a sedative and antidepressant, and it is now being hailed as the herbal answer to Prozac, but of course without the side-effects. The mood-elevating properties can take 2–3 months to produce lasting effects, which are brought about by the plant's ability to enhance the effect of neurotransmitters in the brain. St John's wort increases sensitivity to sunlight and therefore is well worth using to relieve SAD, and may well be helpful for jet lag. It can provide excellent support for emotional problems during the menopause. Taken internally and applied externally, St John's wort is a great remedy for nerve pain and trauma to the nervous system. Some refer to it as "the Arnica of the nerves". It can be thought of for treating trigeminal neuralgia, sciatica, back pain, shingles, headaches and rheumatic pain. The red oil produced when the flowers are macerated in oil in sunlight for two weeks can be applied to sites of nerve pain such as sciatica and shingles, to ease pain and speed healing.

Consult a Professional

Self-help using herbs may well be suitable for straightforward and minor complaints but for more complex and chronic problems, and to enable a greater understanding of specific patterns of health and their treatment, consulting a qualified medical herbalist may well be preferable. After an in depth consultation the practitioner will use his/her skill and expertise to analyse and understand the patient and their

Devil's Claw and Arthritis

A South African herb known as devil's claw (*Harpagophytum procumbens*) enjoyed considerable popularity 20 years ago as a treatment for arthritis. Lacking clinical proof of efficacy, it fell into disuse for that purpose but continued to be valued as an appetite stimulant and a digestive aid.

Now, 8 pharmacologic and 12 clinical reports later (only one of the latter was double-blind, placebo-controlled), the herb is once again gaining some popularity as an anti-inflammatory that reduces pain and allows additional joint flexibility in rheumatoid complaints. If additional clinical studies support the earlier results, devil's claw could become a major player in the treatment of various joint diseases.

Varro E. Tyler, *Prevention*, May 1999.

---

symptoms and to treat accordingly. A herbal prescription, tailor-made to the individual patient is designed to help create the conditions that enable healing. Such a prescription may consist of anything from 1–15 different herbs and will be subject to review during the follow-up consultation. A discussion of diet and lifestyle will also be involved and the practitioner will advise accordingly. People with hormonal imbalances, gynaecological problems and menopausal problems, chronic stress-related symptoms, heart and circulatory disease, skin problems, bowel symptoms such as Crohn's disease and irritable bowel syndrome, as well as chronic infections, would be well advised to consult a medical herbalist. Irritable bowel syndrome is something that crops up in herbal practice on a regular basis, and is complex because those who suffer this problem may be suffering from stress, anxiety or depression, they may have food intolerances or even candida. Their symptoms need to be distinguished from inflammatory bowel problems such as ulcerative colitis and Crohn's disease, infectious enteritis and diverticular disease before treatment is commenced. Treatment will involve changes in eating patterns, elimination of suspect foods such as wheat and dairy products, support for the nervous system and restoring normal bowel function. A herbal prescription may consist of anti-spasmodic and relaxing herbs such as chamomile, hops and lemon balm which are specific for stress-related digestive problems, intended to relieve intestinal spasms, expel gas and relieve pain, combined with nerve tonics, such as skullcap or vervain, with a demulcent remedy such as marshmallow, and the addition of a little peppermint. Psyllium seeds may also be prescribed to regulate bowel function.

Those who are attracted to trying herbal medicine in one form or another are very often people with a love of plants and flowers and a respect for the miraculous world of nature, or they may simply be referred to a remedy or a practitioner by personal recommendation. It is interesting that as gardening continues to be one of the most popular leisure pursuits in this country, even if as a city dweller one only has a patio, balcony or window box, people are increasingly growing herbs. Fascinated not only by their attractive shapes and colours, delicious tastes and often wonderful scents, there is something that people find about growing or being among herbs in the garden that has a subtle healing effect of its own. Just try gazing at a rose and see what happens!

"Most consumers seem to be oblivious to the potentially significant health risks associated with the use of herbal medicines."

Herbal Supplements Can Be Harmful

John M. Allen

John M. Allen argues in the following viewpoint that herbal supplements are potentially hazardous to human health. He contends that many herbs cause hepatitis and other liver problems, cataracts, and cancer. Moreover, according to Allen, herbal supplements are not subjected to the same rigorous tests as are pharmaceutical drugs, so consumers of herbal remedies risk ingesting inappropriate dosages or impure products. Allen maintains that consumers should be aware of the serious risks associated with herbal supplements. Allen is an associate professor in the Department of Chemistry at Indiana State University in Terre Haute.

As you read, consider the following questions:
1. How does the author define herbal medicines and dietary supplements?
2. According to Allen, what is an organic substance?
3. In the author's opinion, how are users of herbal supplements acting as human guinea pigs?

Herbal medicines and dietary supplements represent a booming multibillion-dollar business in the U.S. and around the globe. The herbal medicine phenomenon is part of a much larger "alternative medicine" movement whose proponents seek to exploit both traditional methods of disease prevention and treatment as well as a variety of New Age approaches. There is no question that the active ingredients in some herbal preparations show much promise in the prevention and treatment of a wide variety of illnesses; this is evidenced by a large body of scientific data that has been amassed and published in reputable scientific and medical journals. However, the use of herbal medicines and dietary supplements also poses significant health risks. These risks are largely due to the widely varying nature of herbal preparations and, in the U.S., to the lack of consumer protection ordinarily accorded to drug substances by the Food and Drug Administration (FDA) because herbal medicines and dietary supplements are not officially classified as drugs.

What Are Herbal Supplements?

Herbal medicines and dietary supplements are typically processed plant materials or solvent extracts (essential oils) of plant materials. All plants, including herbs, naturally synthesize many (sometimes hundreds) of complex chemical compounds as part of their metabolic activities. Many of these compounds are not directly related to the plant's energy production but are toxins synthesized by the plant in order to ward off other plants, herbivores, and plant parasites. Thus, all plant materials contain large numbers of chemical compounds, some of which may exert a desired physiological effect and others which may exert no effect whatever or any number of undesirable effects when consumed by humans. In fact, many herbs contain chemical compounds that act oppositely from the principal active ingredient.

In addition to the issue of heterogeneity resulting from plant biosynthesis of large numbers of chemical compounds, it has also been reported that herbal medicines are occasionally contaminated with pesticides, herbicides, heavy metals, microorganisms, and mold toxins, and have occasionally been spiked with other drugs. The chemical composition of many herbal preparations that are sold to consumers is essentially unknown. This situation is tantamount to the consumer of herbal preparations playing chemical Russian roulette. However, the FDA cannot take legal action to restrict the use of a given herbal medicine or dietary supplement until substantial harm has been proven.

Herbal medicines are, in some ways, like illicit street drugs. When a drug user buys crack cocaine or heroin on the street-corner, the dealer has no idea what is really in the glassine envelope or plastic vial and neither does the trafficker who supplies the local dealer. When a consumer buys herbal remedies at a local pharmacy, his or her pharmacist and the company that supplied them to the pharmacy have only limited information as to what is in them; in many cases the supplier merely repackages and distributes these products and pockets a hefty markup. As with street drugs, the dosage and purity of herbal medicines are unknown. However, the effects upon the human body produced by the active ingredients in many herbal medicines are not as well understood as the effects of cocaine or heroin.

The New Age Mantra: Organic and Natural Is Better

The terms "organic" and "natural" have found widespread use in a seemingly infinite variety of contexts. Organic gardening and natural foods come to mind at once. Advertisers frequently claim that their products are "totally organic or one hundred percent natural." What exactly do these phrases mean? Most consumers are convinced through advertising that organic or natural products are intrinsically safer and more effective than synthetic or "chemical" products.

To the average consumer, organic means "good" because synthetic chemicals are "bad"; natural means "wholesome," and anything else is probably loaded with chemicals (i.e., bad). In flyers, some products are even labeled "chemical free." This, of course, is impossible since even the empty product container has air in it which is composed of chemicals. All of this confusion is the result of New Age propaganda and superstition as well as a certain amount of fear of chemicals. Part of the problem is that the word chemical is so frequently used in conjunction with pollution or carcinogen. This results in consumer confusion and anxiety and is exploited by those who derive income from the sale of so-called organic or natural products.

Unfounded and irrational fears of chemicals have been amplified by clever natural food and herbal medicine advertising campaigns to such an extent that many consumers now fear pharmaceutical drugs. So-called natural remedies are touted as safer and healthier alternatives to synthetic chemical pills dispensed from the local pharmacy. There is no evidence to support this proposition; in fact the evidence suggests the opposite conclusion. There is no doubt that many pharmaceutical drugs produce a variety of adverse side effects, but this is also true for herbal remedies. Of course, the rates of incidence and severity of side effects associated with the use of herbal medicines are known mainly through anecdotal evidence, although well-documented reports of serious adverse side effects are becoming more frequent.

At any of the wonderful upscale book and coffee shops at local malls across America and probably in Europe as well, there are entire sections of the magazine racks devoted to extolling the glories of the healing power of herbal medicines and dietary supplements and several shelves of books devoted to the same topics. A little time spent surfing the Internet is both instructive and disturbing. Web pages devoted to such pseudosciences as astrology, rolfing, crystal therapy, colon hydrotherapy, and electromagnetic therapy provide links to other Web sites devoted to the healing power of "natural" herbs and "organic" dietary supplements. One can even buy "pyramid energized" herbs that are supposedly more efficacious because they have been stored under a pyramid. Of course, this powerful effect said to be exerted by pyramids is not really surprising since some claim that storing razor blades under a pyramid keeps them sharp indefinitely. . . .

What Is Organic and Natural?

To a chemist, an organic substance is any substance that contains carbon atoms, and a natural product is simply one derived from plant or animal sources. It is really not possible to determine the meaning of the term "natural" as it is used in the popular literature and in advertising. Morphine that is extracted from opium poppies and morphine that is prepared synthetically are both organic chemical compounds because they both contain carbon atoms. However, there is absolutely no difference between natural morphine extracted from opium poppies and morphine that has been prepared synthetically from bottles of chemicals sitting on a shelf in the laboratory.

There is also absolutely no reason to believe that exposure to naturally derived chemicals is any less likely to be toxic than exposure to synthetic chemicals. For example, a completely natural organic compound called aflatoxin is synthesized by certain fungi that grow on improperly stored corn, peanuts, and plant materials such as herbs. Aflatoxin is thousands of times more toxic to humans than DDT, a much feared synthetic pesticide; it is also a very potent carcinogen (cancer-causing substance).

Reports of Herbal Medicine Toxicity in Medical Literature

Most reports of toxic effects due to the use of herbal medicines and dietary supplements are associated with hepatotoxiciry (liver toxicity) although reports of other toxic effects including kidney, nervous system, blood, cardiovascular, and dermatologic effects, mutagenicity, and carcinogenicity have also been published in the medical literature. The involvement of herbal medicines in kidney toxicity is observed so frequently that it is referred to as Chinese herb nephropathy (CHN) in the medical literature, a progressive form of renal fibrosis.

The risks of toxic effects associated with the use of herbal medicines vary significantly from person to person. "Certain users of herbs are at high risk of intoxication. These include chronic users, those consuming large amounts of a great variety, the very young, fetuses, the sick, the elderly, the malnourished or undernourished, and those on long-term medication" [according to researcher R.J. Huxtable]. What follows is a small sampling of the many reports of adverse health effects associated with the use of herbal medicines and dietary supplements found in the current medical literature.

Herbal preparations containing germander were withdrawn from the market after their use for weight control caused a hepatitis epidemic. Mint tea containing pennyroyal oil (menthofuran and pulegone) was reported to be responsible for the death of one infant and serious injury in another due to hepatic and neurologic injuries. Herb mixtures containing chaparral, aristolchia, ma-huang, germander, and Jin-bu-huan were reported to have produced life-threatening neurologic and cardiovascular manifestations after a single dose in a child, and long-term use in adults has been associated with hepatitis.

St. John's Wort is a very popular over-the-counter herbal preparation used as an antidepressant. The active ingredient in St. John's Wort is a chemical compound called hypericin. Other chemical compounds present in St. John's Wort preparations, their concentrations, and human toxicities are essentially unknown and can vary widely depending upon the source of the herb and subsequent handling. Hypericin, however, absorbs certain frequencies of light and, when present in the eye after oral ingestion of St. John's Wort, can result in alterations of lens proteins that can lead to cataract formation. This observation is indirectly supported by a recently published report in which hypericin was found to produce phototoxic effects in cells. Hypericin passes the light energy that it absorbs to oxygen molecules forming toxic species including free radicals which can subsequently attack and damage a variety of biomolecules. . . .

Use of Herbal Medicines and Increased Risks of Cancers

Pyrrolizidine alkaloids present in comfrey tea and other plant materials are widely recognized as hepatotoxins. In addition, these compounds have been identified as carcinogens. In an animal study done with Russian comfrey leaves and roots on rats, hepatocellular adenomas (a type of liver cancer) were induced in animals that received diets containing comfrey roots and leaves and, less frequently, hemangioendothelial sarcomas (cancer) of the liver were also observed. In a study conducted in the Philippines, users of herbal medicines were found to have elevated risk (2.5 times) of nasopharyngeal carcinomas (nasal and sinus cancers) versus non-users. This effect is thought to occur through the ability of some herbal medications to reactivate the Epstein-Barr vitus (EBV) or through a direct promoting effect upon EBV-transformed cells. Another study found a 49-fold increase in nasopharyngeal carcinomas among those testing positive for EBV who also use herbal medicines. Thus, patients infected with EBV might well want to avoid some herbal remedies in particular. . . .

Herbal Medicine Risks and Human Longevity

Proponents of the use of herbal medicines have argued that these preparations have been used for a long time and that any serious toxicity problems would have been identified by now. This argument is wholly without merit. Herbal remedies have been used for hundreds of years but their toxicities (and in particular their cancer-causing abilities) have, as yet, remained largely unquantified. Even some pharmaceutical drugs that have undergone extensive testing (e.g., thalidomide) have later been found to exert unanticipated toxic effects. One of the most frustrating aspects of studying chemical carcinogenesis is the long latency period between chemical exposure and the development of cancers. This is problematic because it is very difficult to make connections between specific chemical exposures and cancer risks since people are exposed to so many different chemical compounds during their lifetimes. Furthermore, many people who use herbal medicines use more than one herbal preparation. Thus, there are many difficulties posed by multiple exposures over long periods of time in unravelling cancer etiology. Another obstacle to identifying cancer etiologies are the unquantified effects upon carcinogenesis associated with heredity; some people are just more susceptible to certain cancers than others.

Herbal medicines have found widespread use in China for centuries. If the life expectancy in China, let's say, two hundred years ago was short (e.g., thirty years), most people would have died from other causes before they had lived long enough to develop cancers as the result of chemical exposures such as herb ingestion. Furthermore, for most of the past two hundred years, there has been no systematic public health surveillance of human cancers. Thus, if as it appears that some herbal medicines are carcinogenic, we will not observe the effects upon cancer morbidity and mortality rates for several years in the U.S. assuming that widespread use of herbal medicines began ten to fifteen years ago. . . .

The Modern Drug Discovery and Approval Process

When a natural product such as an herb appears to have some desirable medicinal property based upon anecdotal evidence, an investigation of the chemical constituents of the plant material may be conducted. The first step is frequently to prepare a solvent extract of the plant material. When an extract is prepared from a particular medicinal herb, the plant material is dried, pulverized, and boiled in an organic solvent such as methylene chloride with collection and recycling of the solvent vapor in an apparatus that somewhat resembles a still. The solvent is removed and an extract or oil remains. This oil may contain hundreds or thousands of individual chemical compounds. In the case of many medicinal herbs, one or two of these chemical compounds may exert the desired physiological effect. The other compounds present in the extract may be inert, or cause any number of toxic effects when ingested by humans.

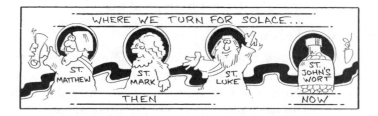

Kauffmann. © 2003 by Joel Kauffmann. Reprinted with permission.

The extract is then carefully fractionated by chromatographic separation methods. Chromatographic separations involve distributing the mixture of chemical compounds extracted from the plant material between a stationary bed of solid particles and a flowing solvent. Under the appropriate conditions, each chemical component (or a fraction containing a small number of chemical components) will migrate through the bed of solid particles at a different rate. Each fraction is collected individually as it reaches the end of the particle bed.

Each fraction is then tested for the desired activity (usually on mice or other small animals). When a fraction is found to have a desired effect, the components in that fraction are subjected to further separation. These more finely separated fractions are then tested for activity. Ultimately, the goal is to identify a specific chemical compound present in the original plant extract that exerts the desired physiological effect.

Once the active chemical compound has been identified, its molecular structure must be determined. This is done by such techniques as nuclear magnetic resonance (NMR) spectroscopy. When the structure of the molecule (i.e., the way in which all of the atoms in the molecule are connected to one another) is mapped out, a synthetic scheme is worked out to build the molecule from scratch. Scratch, in this context, means readily available chemical reagents. Since a given drug molecule may contain as many as a hundred atoms or more, this can be a complex undertaking. Once the synthetic scheme is worked out, the drug is synthesized and purified. The resulting synthetically produced drug is absolutely identical to the drug derived from plant material.

Rigorous Testing

Once the synthetic drug has undergone rigorous assessments of its safety and efficacy as per FDA regulations and is found to be acceptable, it is approved for use by the public. The manufacture of the synthetic drug is strictly regulated by the FDA. Every step is carefully assessed and contaminants are quantified and reduced to a specified concentration level in the final product. This process sometimes takes a very long time and requires the expenditure of vast sums of money by pharmaceutical companies. Once the drug is marketed, reports of any previously unrecognized side effects are monitored by the FDA. If it becomes clear that the use of a given drug represents an unacceptable risk of unwanted side effects, its use may be restricted.

This procedure contrasts quite sharply with the situation regarding herbal preparations. There is rarely any attempt to isolate the active ingredient (if one is actually present) from the herbal plant material or herbal extracts. The presence of deliberately added adulterants (i.e., drugs) and accidental contaminants in the herb or herbal extract is always a risk when these products are not properly tested for purity. However, it should be pointed out that some manufacturers of herbal medicines and dietary supplements do conduct testing in order to assure that their products do not contain deliberately added impurities or accidental contaminants. This testing may also involve determination and standardization of the concentration of an active ingredient. Of course, product testing for purity and standardization of dosage is essentially voluntary and is only conducted by the most reputable manufacturers and distributors. As pointed out previously, many herbal toxicity issues are associated with the chemical compounds that are present in the herb itself rather than deliberately added or accidental contaminants. Thus, when testing for purity is performed, it provides only a limited assurance of safety. . . .

Ingesting Unknown Substances

It is worth repeating that some herbal medicines have demonstrated efficacy for the treatment or prevention of a variety of illnesses. However, in many cases, equally effective and much safer pharmaceutical drugs are available. The consumer of pharmaceutical drugs ingests very well characterized chemical substances while the consumer of herbal medicines and dietary supplements ingests substances of essentially unknown chemical composition. If the use of a given herbal medicine or dietary supplement causes injury to consumers, it may take a long time for this to become apparent, particularly regarding carcinogenicity. Thus, each consumer of herbal preparations is acting as a sort of human guinea pig in a poorly controlled drug study; if enough of them are injured, the FDA can act to protect the rest. Furthermore, successful recovery for damages on behalf of injured consumers may be difficult or impossible.

I do not wish to suggest that the sale of herbal medicines and dietary supplements should be subject to legal prohibitions; it is my position that each individual person should be free to assess the risks and rewards of ingesting chemical substances and act accordingly. However, most consumers seem to be oblivious to the potentially significant health risks associated with the use of herbal medicines and dietary supplements.

Finally, for patients stricken with AIDS or cancer, waiting for the wheels of science, industry, and government to identify, develop, and approve new drugs may not be an option. For these patients, the use of herbal medicines and dietary supplements as well as experimental drugs that have undergone only limited testing may be justified. For the average relatively healthy person, however, the ingestion of herbal medicines and dietary supplements represents the assumption of unquantified, but potentially serious, health risks and dubious benefits.

*"Lack of religious involvement has an effect
on mortality that is equivalent to 40 years
of smoking one pack of cigarettes per day."*

Religious Faith Is Associated with Good Health

Gregg Easterbrook

According to Gregg Easterbrook in the following viewpoint, people who identify themselves as religious and regularly attend worship services experience lower levels of heart disease, cancer, depression, have fewer strokes, and live longer than nonreligious people. Researchers have examined the correlation between faith and health for decades, he reports, and have yet to determine why religion has such a positive effect on a person's health. Among the many theories explaining the faith-health link, according to Easterbrook, is that spirituality confers mental well-being on the believer, and mental well-being is associated with good physical health. Easterbrook is a contributor to the *New Republic*, a magazine of politics and culture.

As you read, consider the following questions:
1. Why are many people in the medical community disturbed by studies that profess a faith-health link, according to Easterbrook?
2. What are "confounders," as defined by the author?
3. According to the author, what is the "good life" movement?

Traditionally, religion is viewed as a haven for the sick and afflicted; Jesus, when he walked the ancient Holy Land, often ministered first to the diseased. But what if the traditional view is wrong and belief actually promotes better health? To the exasperation of some academics, that is what a growing body of medical research is beginning to show.

Recent studies indicate that men and women who practice in any of the mainstream faiths have above-average longevity, fewer strokes, less heart disease, less clinical depression, better immune-system function, lower blood pressure, and fewer anxiety attacks, and they are much less likely to commit suicide than the population at large. These findings come from secular medical schools and schools of public health. The results seem to hold even when researchers control for such variables as believers' health histories, the self-selection effect (whether the kind of people who bound out of bed for a Sabbath service tend to be more able-bodied to begin with), and "social support" (the fact that religious groups offer care networks to those who fall ill). In the most striking finding, Dr. Harold Koenig of Duke University Medical Center has calculated that, with regard to any mainstream faith, "[l]ack of religious involvement has an effect on mortality that is equivalent to 40 years of smoking one pack of cigarettes per day."

Rewards for Attending Service

Koenig and a group of researchers affiliated with such schools as Duke, Harvard, and Yale recently reviewed some 1,100 health-effects studies involving religious practice and found that most, though not all, show statistically significant relationships between worship-service attendance and improved health. (Researchers use service attendance as their proxy because it is an objective data point, as opposed to trying to classify what people privately believe.) In one study, the blood of regular worshipers contained low levels of interleukin-6, a protein associated with immune problems (low is good for interleukin-6). Even subjects with the AIDS virus who regularly practiced a faith had reduced levels of this protein. Another study found that, in Jerusalem, secular Israeli adults "had a significantly higher risk" of heart disease than practicing religious adults.

A 28-year cohort study of approximately 5,000 Californians, conducted by the researcher William Strawbridge and published [in 1997] in the *American Journal of Public Health*, found that women who attended one worship service per week significantly extended their life spans, though benefits were not as clear for men. Strawbridge found that believers as a group were not initially healthier than average (that is, self-selecting and leaving the bedridden behind) but instead tended to start off in worse-than-average health and then gradually improve to superior outcomes. Another new study, conducted mainly by researchers at the University of Texas, found that those who regularly attended worship services lived an average of seven years longer than those who never attended.

Duke's Koenig says the association between religious participation and good health holds for almost all Christianity and Judaism, and he assumes it would hold for Islam as well, though studies have not included enough Muslim subjects to be sure. "The main distinction seems to be whether you are a regular practitioner," Koenig says. "Within Christianity there is very little difference in outcomes among the various denominations, except for nonmainstream denominations. Between Judaism and Christianity there is very little difference." Positive results can pass between generations, too. When parents regularly attend worship services, they increase the odds that their children will live longer, healthier lives.

For nonmainstream denominations, the story is different. Christian Scientists suffer some of the nation's worst longevity statistics, despite their denomination's claim to exalt health. The Faith Assembly, a Christian offshoot whose members may shun medical care, has horrible mortality figures. And when people join cults their health indicators fall off the bottom of the curve. . . .

Suspicion in the Medical Community

Some in the medical community are unhappy about proliferation of studies suggesting a faith-health link or about the fact that 60 of the nation's 126 medical schools now have religion courses on their curricula, a much higher figure than a few years ago. Dr. Richard Sloan of Columbia University's medical school says, "The majority of these studies focus on Christians, suggesting a Christian political agenda behind the work." Even Dr. David Larson, the president of the National Institute for Healthcare Research and a leading exponent of faith-and-medicine—his letterhead proclaims, "Bridging the gap between spirituality and health"—notes, "There is a fair concern this research will be misused by the Christian right." But any U.S. research would have to focus on Christians, since they compose the country's predominant religious group. If there really is a faith-health link, patients deserve to know.

John Billings, the Civil War-era surgeon general of the Army and, later, the first librarian of the New York Public Library, wrote that religion appeared to reduce mortality in the groups he studied. But correlation never proves causation; the fact that people practice a faith and also improve their well-being doesn't establish that religion was the reason.

Medical research is replete with "confounders," complications that can never really be controlled out of studies, no matter how hard researchers try. To cite a mundane example, for decades studies of caffeine have landed all over the map—some find it dangerous, some beneficial, some neutral. Caffeine studies are confounded by the huge range of other influences to which every person is exposed: different diets, lifestyle habits, home and work circumstances, heredity. Researchers try to get confounders to "wash out" of studies by examining large cohorts and also by following subjects for long periods, on the theory that whatever persists is statistically strong. But, even so, it is not unusual for two equally well-done studies to reach widely differing conclusions. If medicine still can't be sure whether a cup of Starbucks helps or hurts, it can't be sure about church, mosque, or synagogue, either.

Examining the Faith-Health Link

Why would practicing a faith improve your longevity and well-being? When studies first began to show a faith-health relationship, many assumed social support would be the explanation. It's clearly an important factor: people who regularly attend religious services are seen by concerned friends who will notice if something appears wrong, call to check up if a person suddenly stops attending, visit, and provide care and encouragement during illness. All these influences improve health and longevity. Merely having a support group that expresses concern if something seems wrong and encourages treatment can be a big plus, as early therapy is almost always most effective.

Public Support for the Health Benefits of Faith

Religious practices such as prayer represent the most prevalent complementary and alternative therapies in the United States. Eighty-two percent of Americans believe in the healing power of personal prayer, 73% believe that praying for someone else can help cure their illness, and 77% believe that God sometimes intervenes to cure people who have a serious illness. A number of studies suggest that spiritual/religious beliefs and practices may contribute to decreased stress and increased sense of well-being, decreased depressive symptoms, decreased substance abuse, faster recovery from hip replacements, improved recovery from myocardial infarction, and enhanced immune system functioning. A . . . meta-analysis of 29 earlier studies involving nearly 126,000 patients argued that the odds of survival were significantly greater for people who scored higher on measures of religious involvement than for people who scored lower, even after controlling for a variety of social and health-related variables, although the design and interpretation of these findings have been questioned.

Linda L. Barnes, Gregory A. Plotnikoff, Kenneth Fox, and Sarah Pendleton, *Pediatrics*, October 2000.

But studies tend to find a faith-health link even when social support is factored out. Some researchers thought the faith-health relationship might emanate from denominational bans against alcohol, caffeine, and smoking or from dietary standards such as the kosher laws. But confound those confounders—it now looks as if small amounts of alcohol might be good for you, while studies don't show much health-benefit distinction between self-denying Seventh Day Adventists and anything-goes Episcopalians.

Current thinking tends toward the assumption that spiritual practice confers its main health benefit by promoting a sensible lifestyle. Specifics differ, but every mainstream Western denomination encourages the flock to drink in moderation, shun drugs, stop smoking, live circumspectly, practice monogamy, get married, and stay married. (Bickering and skillet-throwing notwithstanding, as a group married adults have better health indicators than singles of comparable ages, in part because spouses serve as each other's "social support.") The lifestyle choices encouraged by faith for reasons of theology aren't terribly different from the choices physicians encourage for reasons of playing the percentages. Of course, secular systems of life philosophy also encourage people to practice moderation and fidelity. But, encompassing millions of members and calling on an ultimate authority, religions may simply be doing a better job of advocating the circumspect life, thus conferring comparative health advantages on practitioners.

The believer's lifestyle might even have a historical foundation in the relationship between spiritual practice and longevity. Historians, for instance, are reasonably confident that the Jewish-Muslim prohibition against pork consumption had its origin in protecting believers from trichinosis. Perhaps self-preservation effects such as this extend across many aspects of religion. Those faiths that taught adherents to live circumspectly and care for one another were more likely to prosper, passing down their assumptions, and their health benefits, to the present day.

Spiritual Selection

Jumping off from that, Dr. Herbert Benson of Harvard Medical School has proposed that one reason faith may be linked to better health—indeed, a reason faith and society are historically linked—is that natural selection favors religion. In Benson's theory, during prehistory those clans or groups that possessed the stirrings of religious belief would have developed better health habits and recognized a responsibility to care for family and neighbors. This would have increased "kin fitness," or the likelihood that the group overall would pass along its members' genes. Descendants were then raised with a disposition toward belief; the descendants increased their own survival fitness through faith-motivated health habits and altruistic care of others; they created new descendants and so on. In this way, Benson thinks, human beings became "wired for God," genetically predisposed to have faith. Obviously, religion did not confer a selection advantage in every case: sometimes it caused communities to become targets of war or to engage in internal repression. But, on the macroscale of evolution, those who believed were likelier to live long, healthy lives than those who did not believe. The same, Benson thinks, remains true today.

None of the respectable faith-and-health researchers proposes that religion extends longevity through supernatural agency. Some do, however, take seriously the utility of prayer. Studies of "intercessionary" prayer—Person A prays for the health of Person B—haven't turned up much. But studies do suggest that prayer favorably influences health outcomes for the person who does the praying.

The nonsectarian form of prayer that is akin to meditation has long been recognized by clinicians to improve composure and the sense of well-being; anyone can benefit from a period of meditative prayer each day. Studies at Duke University and elsewhere have recently found that traditional religious "petitionary" prayer, or silently addressing God, also favors health. In one study, subjects who both attended worship services and regularly prayed had lower blood pressure than the control group. Researchers assume that traditional prayer can confer health benefits through the psychological effects of equanimity. Benson's studies, for instance, suggest that a calm state of mind improves the body's self-healing abilities.

Camps in the medical community were displeased when the American Cancer Society recently declared, "Sometimes answers come from prayer when medical science has none." On one level the statement is inarguable; reverence for higher purpose might comfort the victim of illness in ways that no drug or technology ever could. But conventional medicine is comfortable only with the sociological notion that the sick may console themselves by addressing a Maker, real or speculative. The idea that there is an actual reply, that "answers come from prayer," is one that makes much of the medical establishment uneasy, even if the source of the "answer" is no more than the person's own contemplative understanding.

Yet one of the modern era's little secrets is that it is hardly only the Bible-thumpers who pray. John Houghton, among the world's foremost atmospheric physicists and a leading proponent of global-warming theory, regularly prays and has written articles on the value of prayer. The Nobel Prize–winning physicist Charles Townes, principal inventor of the laser beam, says that he prays daily. Pundits might snicker, but, if regular prayer composes the mind and confers health benefits, the person who prays is following the intelligent course, regardless of the verity of any religion.

Mental Health

Another possibility for the link between longevity and faith turns on mental health. Koenig suspects that many physical benefits of religious practice originate with the sense of well-being or purposefulness that believers report: he finds it revealing that the faithful experience fewer bouts of clinical depression than the population at large and that, when depression does strike, they recover faster. In this view, faith doesn't merely have an agreeable placebo effect on the mind but helps believers acquire coping mechanisms that ward off stress and anxiety, lower stress in turn being favorable for physical health. Dr. Esther Steinberg, a researcher at the National Institute of Mental Health, devotes a fine new book, *A Delicate Balance*, to the evidence that health and quality of life are improved by possessing an affirmative emotional sense, including the belief that existence is worthwhile and has purpose.

The mental health point isn't just a detached observation. Sternberg's premise, after all, is not much different from saying that postmodernism is bad for your health. Many in the academic establishment are uncomfortable with evidence that belief promotes mental health, as this implies that faith ought to be the normative condition, compared to unbelief.

Here faith-and-health treads some of the same ground as the emerging "good life" movement in psychology. Postwar psychology and social science have emphasized dysfunction, studying what causes people to become alienated or antisocial. The good-life movement seeks instead to emphasize what causes people to become high-minded and altruistic. "Good life" in this sense means the admirable path, not wine and roses; Eleanor Roosevelt is a favorite topic of good-life proponents. Martin Seligman of the University of Pennsylvania, recently president of the American Psychological Association, is a leader in this evolving discipline, having said that scholars ought to "turn their eyes to the best in life."

The regnant intellectual view is that the awful truth about society is revealed when people are driven to madness; the good-life movement asserts, instead, that the shining truth is revealed when people become selfless. But academia is today much more comfortable with lamenting ugliness than endorsing virtue. To hold up Eleanor Roosevelt—anyone else— as a psychological archetype goes against the current vogue for radical nonjudgmentalism.

A New Argument for Faith

There's an obvious corollary here between good-life psychology and the faith-and-health question. If psychology ought to be focusing on what causes morality, and mainstream religions promote morality and mental health, we have a new argument for taking faith seriously. The cynical view of religion was so deeply ingrained in postwar intellectual thought that, until 1994, the American Psychiatric Association classified strong spiritual belief as a "disorder." Now faith is looking like a health boon. Quite a switcheroo.

And, speaking of fun twists, it's established that physicians have an obligation to advise patients to take steps that research shows to be associated with longevity, such as not smoking. It's also established that doctors may counsel patients on highly personal subjects, such as sexual behavior. So, if faith increases your odds of good health, does this mean your physician has an obligation to advise you to become religious?

Sloan, of Columbia, says he fears doctors may soon be pressured to dispense such advice and counters that, although research has shown that being married correlates with better health, this does not cause physicians to advise patients to rush to the chapel. The trouble with this reasoning is that counseling patients to wed is not utilitarian: there's no guarantee you'll find a compatible partner. Recommending religion, on the other hand, is quite pragmatic advice. Anyone can join a faith; attending services is a lot easier than quitting smoking.

Nevertheless, "Even if the research shows that religion is good for health, that doesn't mean doctors should prescribe it like antibiotics," says Larson, the faith-and-health advocate. Koenig thinks the research only demonstrates that physicians should "ask the patient if he or she practices a religion and, if so, what the physician can do to offer support. At this point, we have enough research to say that is good clinical medicine."

Spiritual awareness may indeed be good for you, but it's just as well that your doctor not double as clergy. If faith ever became a formal adjunct of medicine, HMOs could end up publishing lists of preferred-provider churches, mosques, and synagogues, requiring a precertification number before the priest can perform last rites, and—well, you can guess the rest.

"The evidence of an association between religion, spirituality, and health is weak and inconsistent."

Religious Faith Has Not Been Proven to Promote Good Health

Richard P. Sloan, Emilia Bagiella, and Tia Powell

In the following viewpoint Richard P. Sloan, Emilia Bagiella, and Tia Powell contend that research claiming a link between religion and good health is misleading. The authors allege that most studies finding a faith-health link have failed to control for important variables, such as the age, sex, and health status of the participants. Thus, they contend that attending church has no proven health benefits. Sloan is the director of the Behavioral Medicine Program at Columbia-Presbyterian Medical Center in New York. Bagiella is an assistant professor of clinical biostatistics at Columbia University, and Powell is the director of clinical ethics at Columbia-Presbyterian Medical Center.

As you read, consider the following questions:

1. According to the authors, why do Roman Catholic priests have lower rates of morbidity and mortality than nonreligious people?
2. Why do the authors contend that it is harmful to promote faith as an adjunctive medical treatment?
3. How does religious affiliation differ from other factors that affect health, such as smoking, in the authors' opinion?

Richard P. Sloan, Emilia Bagiella, and Tia Powell, "Religion, Spirituality, and Medicine," *Lancet*, vol. 353, February 20, 1999, p. 664. Copyright © 1999 by The Lancet Publishing Group. Reproduced by permission.

R eligion and science share a complex history as well as a complex present. At various times worldwide, medical and spiritual care was dispensed by the same person. At other times, passionate (even violent) conflicts characterised the association between religion and medicine and science. As interest in alternative and complementary medicine has grown, the notion of linking religious and medical interventions has become widely popular, especially in the USA. For many people, religious and spiritual activities provide comfort in the face of illness. However, as US medical schools increasingly offer courses in religion and spirituality and as reports continue to indicate interest in this subject among both physicians and the general public, it is essential to examine how, if at all, medicine should address these issues. Here, in a comprehensive, though not systematic, review of the empirical evidence and ethical issues we make an initial attempt at such an examination.

Interest in Connecting Religion and Medicine

In a recent poll of 1000 US adults, 79% of the respondents believed that spiritual faith can help people recover from disease, and 63% believed that physicians should talk to patients about spiritual faith. Recent articles in such US national newspapers as the *Atlanta Constitution*, *Washington Post*, *Chicago Tribune*, and *USA Today* report that religion can be good for your health. A new magazine, *Spirituality and Health*, edited by the former editor of *Harvard Business Review*, has begun publication. [Researcher D.M.] Eisenberg and colleagues, in a widely cited article on unconventional therapies, noted that 25% of all respondents reported using prayer as medical therapy. [Researchers D.E.] King and [B.] Bushwick reported that 48% of hospital inpatients wanted their physicians to pray with them.

Within the medical community, there is also considerable interest. Meetings sponsored by the US National Institute of Aging, the National Center for Medical Rehabilitation Research, and the Mind/Body Medical Institute, Beth Israel Deaconess Hospital, Boston, have drawn large, enthusiastic audiences. Nearly 30 US medical schools include in their curricula courses on religion, spirituality, and health. Of 296 physicians surveyed during the October, 1996, meeting of the American Academy of Family Physicians, 99% were convinced that religious beliefs can heal, and 75% believed that prayers of others could promote a patient's recovery. [Author R.H.] Benson writes that faith in God has a health-promoting effect. [Researchers D.B.] Larson and [D.A.] Matthews argue for spiritual and religious interventions in medical practice, hope that the "wall of separation" between medicine and religion will be torn down, and assert that "the medicine of the future is going to be prayer and Prozac." In an American Medical Association publication, Matthews and colleagues recommend that clinicians ask "what can I do to support your faith or religious commitment?" to patients who respond favourably to questions about whether religion or faith are "helpful in handling your illness."

Empirical Evidence

In many studies, religion, as a putative antecedent to health outcomes, has been measured in several ways—eg, assessment of religious behaviours, such as frequency of church attendance or prayer; dimensions of religious experience, such as the comfort it may provide; and health differences as a function of differences in religious denomination or degree of religious orthodoxy.

In addition, health outcomes vary considerably—eg, physical disease outcomes, mental health outcomes, and health behaviours. Here, we consider methodological issues that pertain to studies of physical disease outcomes.

Control for Confounding Variables and Other Covariates

Confounders such as behavioural and genetic differences and stratification variables such as age, sex, education, ethnicity, socioeconomic status, and health status may have an important role in the association between religion and health. Failure to control for these factors can lead to a biased estimation of this association. Multivariate methods allow estimation of the magnitude of the association between religious variables and health outcomes while controlling for the effects of other variables. However, use of these methods requires complete presentation of the results—at least the coefficients and corresponding confidence intervals for all the variables in the statistical model. Reports that fail to do this are incomplete and may be misleading.

Attempts to assess the effect of degree of religiousness on health outcomes show this. Increased religious devotion, assessed as service as a Roman Catholic priest, nun, Morman priest, or Trappist or Benedictine monk, is associated with reductions in morbidity and mortality. These cases, however, were selected for study precisely because they are inclined to stricter adherence to codes of conduct that proscribe behaviours associated with risk (eg, smoking, alcohol consumption, sexual activity, psychosocial stress, and in some cases, consumption of meat).

Is Spirituality Helpful?

A 1996 poll of 1,000 adults found that 79% believed that spiritual faith can help people recover from disease. This idea is also popular among physicians. Although many studies have found associations between various measures of religiosity and health, no well-designed study has demonstrated that religious beliefs or prayer actually benefit health. In fact, one well-designed study found just the opposite. The study involved patients whose progress was followed for nine months after discharge from a British hospital. They evaluated the outpatient records and the responses of 189 patients to questionnaires. The researchers concluded that the health status of patients with stronger spiritual beliefs were more than twice as likely to be unimproved or worse. Although some studies have found that churchgoers tend to be healthier and to live longer than nonchurchgoers, church attendance itself is unlikely to be responsible for the difference.

Stephen Barrett, *Quackwatch*, December 17, 2001.

In a series of studies from Israel, religiousness, measured as religious orthodoxy, was also shown to confer health benefits. However, one of these was a case-control study, the deficiencies of which are widely known. In another, a multivariate model that predicted mortality from coronary heart disease included standard risk factors but omitted religion, and no information on risk-ratio or confidence intervals or even level of statistical significance was provided. Finally, in a study matching secular and religious Kibbutzim according to location, use of the same regional hospital, and members older than 40 years, all-cause mortality was significantly greater among members of the secular Kibbutzim. However, the strategy of matching ensures equivalence of groups only on the matched variables. As a consequence, the groups differed with respect to dietary habits, smoking, blood cholesterol concentrations, and marital status, with the secular group having greater risk, as the authors themselves report. The multivariate analysis of mortality did not control for these factors.

Control for confounding and other covariates also affects studies that report that religious behaviours and experiences influence health outcomes. In some studies with large databases, this problem can be addressed. Both the Alameda County Study and the Tecumseh Community Health Study showed that frequency of attendance at religious services was inversely associated with mortality. However, after control for all relevant covariates, this relation held only for women. In another large study, attendance at religious services was associated with increased functional capacity in the elderly but after control for appropriate covariates, this relation held for only 3 of the 7 years in which outcome data were collected. There was no effect on mortality. In a smaller study, religiousness predicted mortality in the elderly poor but only among those in poor health.

Nonexistent Findings

In many other studies, inadequate control for important covariates points to significant findings when none may exist. For example, [researcher P.] Pressman and colleagues reported that among elderly women after surgical repair of broken hips, religiousness was associated with better ambulation status at discharge. Although the analysis controlled for severity of health condition, it did not control for age, a critical variable when studying functional capacity in the elderly.

In some cases, problems of interpretation arise not so much in the original research but rather in secondary sources. A case in point is a report by [researchers G.W.] Comstock and

[K.B.] Partridge, frequently cited as showing a positive association between church attendance and health. However, as Comstock himself later reported, this finding was probably due to failure to control for the important covariate of functional capacity: people with reduced capacity (and poorer health) were less likely to go to church. This latter study is rarely cited. Similarly [researchers H.G.] Koenig reports that a study by [researcher A.] Colantonio and colleagues "found lower rates of stroke in persons who attended religious services at least once per week . . .". However, this was only the case for the univariate analysis and the effect disappeared after covariates such as levels of physical function were added to the analysis. [Scientist J.S.] Levin, in a review of a review, reported that 22 of 27 studies of religious attendance and health showed a significant positive relation, despite his own previous assertion that associations between attendance and health are highly questionable because this research is characterised by numerous methodological problems including the failure to adjust for confounders and covariates.

Finally, many studies evaluate differences in health indicators as a function of religious denomination. However, they are generally conducted precisely because religious groups differ on risk behaviours such as smoking and alcohol consumption or on genetic heritage.

Failure to Control for Multiple Comparisons

Many studies on religion and health fail to make an adjustment for the greater likelihood of finding a statistically significant result when conducting multiple statistical tests. For example, one study reported that religious attendance was inversely associated with high concentrations of interleukin-6 [a harmful protein] in the elderly. However, interleukin-6 was one of eight outcome variables and there was no attempt to control for multiple comparisons, as the authors themselves reported. In a retrospective study, the associations between frequency of prayer and six items measuring subjective health were examined. Analyses of variance were conducted on each of these six perceptions of health and three revealed effects of frequency of prayer at the 0.05 level of statistical significance. In such studies, adjustments of levels to control for such multiple comparisons would render these findings non-significant.

There are similar problems in the only published randomised clinical trial. In this double-blind study, patients in a coronary-care unit (CCU) were assigned randomly either to standard care or to daily intercessory prayer ministered by three to seven born-again Christians. Outcome variables were measured, and on six the prayer group had fewer newly diagnosed ailments. However, the six significant outcomes were not independent: the prayer group had fewer cases of newly diagnosed heart failure and of newly prescribed diuretics and fewer cases of newly diagnosed pneumonia and of newly prescribed antibiotics. There was no control for multiple comparisons, a fact recognised by the author. To address this issue, "multivariant" analysis was conducted but the results were not presented, except for a p value for overall model.

Conflicting Findings

Published work on religion and health lacks consistency, even among well-conducted studies. For example, while [researchers E.L.] Idler and [S.V.] Kasl found some effects of religious attendance on functional capacity in the elderly, measures of "religious involvement", an index of the "private, reflective" aspects of religion, were not associated with any health outcome. Neither church attendance nor religious involvement was associated with lower mortality. However, in two other large studies, church attendance was associated with lower mortality, but only in women.

Inconsistencies also arise within studies not based on large epidemiological samples. For instance, when each individual item from the scale of religiousness used by Idler and Kasl, was used in another study, "religious comfort and strength" was significantly associated with lower mortality after cardiac surgery in the elderly even after control for relevant confounders. However, the other items from this scale, including religious attendance, did not predict mortality. Moreover, when the entire scale was used, the relation between religion and mortality failed to reach significance. [Scientist R.C.] Byrd reported an advantage in hospital course for the group receiving prayer compared with the control group. However, the groups did not differ in days in the CCU [Critical Care Unit], length of stay in hospital, and number of discharge medications. While total cholesterol concentrations were lower across all age groups for a cohort of Seventh Day Adventists (SDAs) than in age-matched healthy New York City men and women, suggesting a lower risk of coronary heart disease among SDAs, serum triglycerides of the SDA men in the coronary-prone age range (>32 years) were 19% higher than in the controls, which suggests the opposite.

To some degree, lack of consistency is characteristic of an evolving field and may be the product of differences in study design, definitions of religious and spiritual variables, and outcome variables. The absence of specific definitions of religious and spiritual activity is an important problem, since many of the studies to which we refer define these activities differently. Published research would be substantially improved with better definitions of these terms. However, inconsistency in the empirical findings makes it difficult to support recommendations for clinical interventions.

Ethical Issues

Health professionals, even in these days of consumer advocacy, influence patients by virtue of their medical expertise. When doctors depart from areas of established expertise to promote a non-medical agenda, they abuse their status as professionals. Thus, we question inquiries into a patient's spiritual life in the service of making recommendations that link religious practice with better health outcomes. Is it really appropriate, as Matthews and colleagues recommend, for a physician to ask patients what he or she can do to support their faith or religious commitment?

A second ethical consideration involves the limits of medical intervention. If religious or spiritual factors were shown convincingly to be related to health outcomes, they would join such factors as socioeconomic status and marital status, already well established as significantly associated with health. Although physicans may choose to engage patients in discussions of these matters to understand them better, we would consider it unacceptable for a physician to advise an unmarried patient to marry because the data show that marriage is associated with lower mortality. This is because we generally regard financial and marital matters as private and personal, not the business of medicine, even if they have health implications. There is an important difference between "taking into account" marital, financial, or religious factors and "taking them on" as the objects of interventions.

A third ethical problem concerns the possibility of doing harm. Linking religious activities and better health outcomes can be harmful to patients, who already must confront age-old folk wisdom that illness is due to their own moral failure. Within any individual religion, are the more devout adherents "better" people, more deserving of health than others? If evidence showed health advantages of some religious denominations over others, should physicians be guided by this evidence to counsel conversion? Attempts to link religious and spiritual activities to health are reminiscent of the now discredited research suggesting that different ethnic groups show differing levels of moral probity, intelligence, or other measures of social worth. Since all human beings, devout or profane, ultimately will succumb to illness, we wish to avoid the additional burden of guilt for moral failure to those whose physical health fails before our own.

Some practitioners who link faith and medical practice do so appropriately, and in ways that do not depend on utilitarian expectations of better health. For instance, devout health professionals may view their work as an extension of their religious beliefs. Such physicians may or may not choose to share their opinions with patients. However, some patients and doctors may be aware of a common faith. There is no ethical objection to co-worshippers discussing medical issues in the context of a shared faith. Indeed, a thorough understanding of a patient's religious values can be extremely important in discussing critical medical issues, such as care at the end of life. Irrespective of the practitioner's religion, respectful attention must be paid to the impact of religion on the patient's decisions about health care.

An especially poignant example of the devout practitioner who appropriately notes connections between illness, recovery, and prayers of thanks is provided by [Doctor K.] Prager, in describing a serious illness in his son. Prager does not suggest that his son recovers function because he is faithful, but rather teaches how the faithful may give thanks for recovery. Such connections between faith and health are valuable because they are sensitive to all aspects of the patient's experience, yet in no way depend on spurious claims about scientific data.

Weak Evidence

Even in the best studies, the evidence of an association between religion, spirituality, and health is weak and inconsistent.

We believe therefore that it is premature to promote faith and religion as adjunctive medical treatments. However, between the extremes of rejecting the idea that religion and faith can bring comfort to some people coping with illness and endorsing the view that physicians should actively promote religious activity among patients lies a vast uncharted territory in which guidelines for appropriate behaviour are needed urgently.

Nonetheless, caution is required. There is a temptation to conclude that this matter can be resolved as soon as methodologically sound empirical research becomes available. Even the existence of convincing evidence of a relation between religious activity (however defined) and beneficial health outcomes may not eliminate the ethical concerns that we raise here. Religious pursuits, such as decisions to marry or have children, are qualitatively different from health behaviours such as quitting smoking or eating a low-fat diet, even if they are linked unequivocally to health benefits.

No-one can object to respectful support for patients who draw upon religious faith in times of illness. However, until these ethical issues are resolved, suggestions that religious activity will promote health, that illness is the result of insufficient faith, are unwarranted.

Periodical Bibliography

The following articles have been selected to supplement the diverse views presented in this chapter.

Skye Alexander — "Don't Just Do Something, Sit There," *Better Nutrition*, November 2000.

Marcia Angell and Jerome P. Kassirer — "Alternative Medicines: The Risks of Untested and Unregulated Remedies," *Skeptical Inquirer*, January/February 1999.

Benjamin J. Ansell — "When 'Health' Supplements May Do Harm," *New York Times*, September 17, 2002.

Cary Barbor — "The Science of Meditation," *Psychology Today*, May 2001.

Stephen Barrett — "Acupuncture, Qigong, and 'Chinese Medicine,'" *Quackwatch*, September 22, 2002.

Carrie Bodane and Kenneth Brownson — "The Growing Acceptance of Complementary and Alternative Medicine," *Health Care Manager*, March 2002.

Sidney Callahan — "Alternative Treatment: Maybe Snake Oil Works," *Commonweal*, November 5, 1999.

Larry Dossey — "Prayer Is Good Medicine: The Evidence for Spiritual Healing Is One of Medical Science's Best-Kept Secrets," *Saturday Evening Post*, November/December 1997.

Diane Guernsey — "My Prayers: While No One Has Definitive Answers, a Personal Journey Sheds Light on This Humble Act and, Surprisingly, on Who Can Benefit from It," *Town & Country*, May 2002.

Carol J. Henderson — "Alternative Treatments Come with Complement of Risks—Though Plentiful, Information on Dietary Supplements Is Confusing and Outcomes Are Not Well Documented," *Biomechanics*, November 1, 2002.

Samuel McCracken — "The New Snake Oil: A Field Guide," *Commentary*, June 1999.

Vojtech Mornstein — "Alternative Medicine and Pseudoscience: Comments of a Biophysicist," *Skeptical Inquirer*, November/December 2002.

David W. Ramey — "The Scientific Evidence of Homeopathy," *Priorities for Health*, 2000.

Patricia Roy

"Hemlock Is Natural Too: Think Twice About Using Alternative Medicines, This Physician Tells Her Patients," *Medical Economics*, November 8, 2002.

George A. Ulett

"Acupuncture, Magic, and Make-Believe," *Skeptical Inquirer*, March/April 2003.

Geoff Watts

"The Power of Nothing: With the Right Encouragement, Your Mind Can Convince the Body to Heal Itself. What Is the Mysterious Force That Conventional Medicine Seems to Have Forgotten?" *New Scientist*, May 26, 2001.

CHAPTER 4

How Can Government Policies Promote Good Health?

Chapter Preface

Many government agencies, such as the Bureau of Alcohol, Tobacco, and Firearms (ATF), strive to protect consumers from the potential health risks that accompany various products. In addition to restricting access to certain items, such as prescription drugs, the government requires that manufacturers inform consumers of the known health risks that are associated with their products. Alcohol manufacturers, for example, are required to attach warning labels to their bottles about the possible health problems associated with drinking. Recently winemakers have argued that the warning labels on bottles of wine should also inform the consumer of the health benefits of drinking wine.

Americans first became aware of the health benefits of wine consumption after *60 Minutes* aired a program on the "French paradox" in 1996. The program showed that the French, despite their high fat diets, have a much lower incidence of coronary heart disease than Americans. Their secret: wine consumption. Since the program aired, scientists have announced that drinking wine offers numerous other health benefits, including a lower risk of stroke, diabetes, kidney stones, high cholesterol, gallbladder disease, Alzheimer's disease, and dementia. Indeed, daily wine drinkers have a 35 percent lower chance of developing heart disease than people who do not drink wine. Moreover, red wine in particular is packed with powerful antioxidants, which are known to reduce the risk of many types of cancer. Wine drinkers also live longer than non–wine drinkers.

In response to these findings the U.S. Department of Agriculture's 1996 *Dietary Guidelines for Americans* suggested that moderate alcohol consumption carried cardiovascular health benefits. The wine industry immediately set about looking for ways to inform the public of the guidelines. Winemakers proposed a federally sanctioned label on wine bottles that would say "To learn about the health effects of wine consumption, consult the *Dietary Guidelines for Americans*." A separate label would advise wine buyers to consult their doctors to learn more about wine and health. According to John De Luca, president of the Wine Institute, a nonprofit organization, "We thought the dietary guidelines were fair and did provide good consumer information."

The ATF approved the proposed labels in 1999. However, the labels caused an uproar among anti-alcohol activists and legislators, who insisted that they would encourage alcohol abuse. The National Council on Alcoholism (NCA) called the labels "potentially disastrous," and South Carolina senator Strom Thurmond stated that the labels "may be seen as the government's endorsement of drinking." Others argued that combining statements that endorsed the health benefits of moderate wine-drinking with warnings of the deleterious health effects of excessive alcohol consumption would confuse the consumer. In response to the backlash the ATF put a moratorium on the labels that remained in place until 2003.

In March 2003 the Alcohol and Tobacco Tax and Trade Bureau (TTB), which took over the label policing duties that used to be handled by the ATF, approved the labels that had been proposed by the wine industry in 1999. However wine bottles had to include the following disclaimer: "This statement should not encourage you to drink or to increase your alcohol consumption for health reasons." According to the TTB, without such a disclaimer, even neutrally worded statements in labeling or advertising "are presumed to be misleading." Many people in the wine industry resent the restrictions on the labels and regard the TTB's policies as censorship. As stated by Sam Kazman, general counsel for the Competitive Enterprise Institute, an advocacy organization that has been active in opposing the rule, "Despite the fact that alcohol's risks are well known, and are prominently stated on every beverage label, [the TTB] is now demanding that these risks be spelled out in even more detail before the public can be told about the health benefits of moderate consumption. In reality, these demands are an attempt to block truthful information that much of the public would find useful. This is paternalistic censorship, pure and simple."

Experts contend that the battle over wine labeling is far from over. Regulations on wine labels is one of many government policies geared toward protecting public health. Authors debate the effectiveness of other public health policies in the following chapter.

"Small incentives to change behavior, such as increasing prices, can have a noticeable effect [on junk-food consumption]."

Junk-Food Taxes May Encourage People to Eat Healthy Foods

Hanna Rosin

In the following viewpoint Hanna Rosin argues that increasing taxes on junk foods may encourage people to purchase healthy fruits and vegetables instead of high-fat, sugary snacks. According to Rosin, researchers have conducted experiments that tested whether people would choose low-priced healthy foods over regular-priced junk foods in vending machines and in high schools. In each experiment, she contends, sales of low-calorie snacks, fruits, and vegetables increased, and sales of unhealthy foods decreased. These experiments, in the author's opinion, suggest that increasing the cost of junk foods may promote healthy food choices. Rosin is a reporter for the *Washington Post*.

As you read, consider the following questions:
1. According to the author, why is regulating fat less intrusive than regulating tobacco?
2. Why do most people consider a fat tax a farfetched idea, in Rosin's opinion?
3. How can the government encourage schools to provide healthier meals, as suggested by the author?

You knew tobacco heavies were getting desperate when they seized on this forgettable quotation, spoken by a Yale professor to the second-string paper in Boston [*The Boston Herald*]: "To me, there is no difference between Ronald McDonald and Joe Camel." Within a week, the quote has found its way into high-decibel opinion columns across the country, and it eventually screeched its way into a prophetic *Wall Street Journal* editorial entitled "Who's Next?" "First, public health groups will determine that hamburgers cause cancer and heart disease," the editorialists warned. "The trial lawyers will begin class actions on behalf of adults who blame their illness on . . . special sauce." Before we know it, poor Ronald McDonald will be doing time for peddling poison to kids, and the rest of us will be reduced to cutting out contraband photos of smoking starlets with those neon-orange safety scissors they hand out in kindergarten.

Slippery Slope Arguments

The *Wall Street Journal*'s reasoning is built on the same assumption as all slippery slope arguments: The human mind is like the canine mind; once legislators get a taste of blood, they won't know where to stop. But the *Journal* is out of luck. The Yale professor, Dr. Kelly Brownell, is not leading a mass movement on the streets of New Haven and has no plans to do so. As director of Yale's Center for Eating and Weight Disorders, Brownell spends his days devising sensible, individually tailored diets for patients who are either wasting away or growing dangerously obese from various food-related obsessions.

True, he's writing a book about how to fix what he calls our "toxic food environment," the publication of which is likely to prompt another alarmist editorial in *The Wall Street Journal*. But, though Brownell has been talking about his ideas for over a decade, so far he's found little enthusiasm for them in the academic community—let alone the wider world. (The normally alarmist Center for Science in the Public Interest calls Brownell's suggestions "pretty extreme.") Most of his data come from only a handful of studies done by the University of Minnesota researchers. And, even on the slowest news day, three professors do not constitute an alarming trend.

It's too bad Brownell isn't more popular. If you accept that America is entering a Puritan phase, then regulating fat can actually be a less intrusive policy than regulating tobacco. Eating habits are more flexible than smoking habits. While people can become addicted to nicotine, they can't become addicted to fat (not medically speaking, at least). By that logic, even small incentives to change behavior, such as increasing prices, can have a noticeable effect.

The Obesity Epidemic

Brownell's reasoning starts with the premise that the number of diet-related deaths is in the same ballpark as the number of tobacco-related deaths: 300,000 a year and climbing for food, compared with 500,000 a year and dropping for smoke. About one-third of the U.S. population is 20 percent or more overweight and is therefore at risk of suffering high cholesterol, high blood pressure, and other cardiovascular diseases. Fat advocates dispute these numbers and will likely argue that Brownell (and I) are shills for the diet industry, but several reputable organizations have independently confirmed the dangers of obesity, including the Centers for Disease Control and the Harvard School of Public Health.

To date, all theories on how to control the epidemic of obesity have failed in practice or even backfired. The scientific pendulum has swung from blaming evil outside forces, to blaming individuals, and back to evil forces again—that is, from blaming Freudian oral fixations, to blaming overindulgent appetites, to blaming bad genes. Brownell wants to stop it somewhere in the middle, to hold people responsible for their own weight loss but help them out a bit. How can anyone lose weight, he argues, when temptation is everywhere, when three new McDonald's restaurants open up every day, when at any hour of the day or night you can treat yourself to a Value Meal from the shame-free anonymity of the drive-thru? "It is tragic," says Brownell, speaking on a cell phone that picks up the clop-clop of the vigorous, fat-melting Yale tennis match he is watching, "that any American child you stop on the street will recognize 'super-size' as a verb."

To nudge people away from the drive-thru, Brownell advocates *The Wall Street Journal's* worst nightmare: a fat tax, where foods with high fat content are taxed at a higher rate. In an ideal world, Brownell would have the government subsidize fruits and vegetables and tax foods with more than a certain number of grams of fat. Carrots should be dirt cheap, he says, but you should have to think twice before buying carrot cake.

Politically Feasible

Small taxes on soft drinks, candy, gum, and snack foods are politically feasible and, when revenues are applied to health programs, are likely to be supported by many consumers. We suggest that public health professionals consider recommending snack taxes as a means of funding healthy eating and physical activity programs. Such programs could result in better health and lower health care costs.

Michael F. Jacobson and Kelly D. Brownell, *American Journal of Public Health*, June 2000.

Most people consider the fat tax a far-fetched idea. Measuring fat content is not always practical. Hamburger meat has a certain percentage of fat, but most of it would melt away during grilling. And what about sugary no-fat snacks such as soda and candy? Besides, a version of the fat tax has already been tried—and it failed. Over the last decade, California, Maryland, and Maine instituted snack taxes levied mostly on junk food such as candy bars, potato chips, and soda. The Snack Food Association eventually killed the tax in all but one state.

Cost Experiments

Short of the tax, though, other experiments with pricing incentives have had a dramatic effect on eating habits. One of the Minnesota researchers, Dr. Robert Jeffery, went to a grocery store to monitor whether customers paid attention to nutrition education posters. After a few days, he realized they noticed the signs, but not nearly as much as they noticed sales. A huge neon cholesterol warning in the dairy section would be totally ignored if eggs were selling at half price that week.

His revelation led to the vending machine experiment. Dr. Jeffery, Dr. Simone French, and some other researchers picked a vending machine at a university and reduced the prices of all products containing less than three grams of fat— pretzels, baked potato chips, Snackwell's foods, rice cakes, animal crackers, granola bars, fat-free fudge—by 50 percent. In three weeks, the percentage of low-fat snacks purchased increased by 80 percent, from 25 percent of total purchases to about 46 percent. Customers purchased many more low-fat snacks, while the sales of fatty snacks decreased modestly.

The researchers then took their experiment to the nutritionist's favorite experimental milieu: high school cafeterias. They picked two high schools—one mostly white, suburban, and middle-class, the other inner-city and ethnically diverse— and discounted salads, bags of carrots, and fruits by 50 percent. After three weeks, nobody bought more salads, but sales of carrots doubled in the suburban school, and sales of fruit quadrupled in the urban school. Total food sales and total number of customers did not change significantly, so the same people must have been substituting healthier foods for their usual choices. . . .

What can we do with these results? They prove, at least, that some form of food tax isn't as regressive as a tobacco tax. True, people with low incomes spend more of their income on food and buy more junk food. But calling the tax regressive assumes it doesn't work. They may have a hard time giving up cigarettes, but it seems relatively easy to convince poor consumers to replace a cookie with an apple.

An Uphill Battle

Of course, nutritionists are fighting an uphill battle. High school cafeterias aren't what they used to be. Most are now mini-malls, where Papa John's pizza and Taco Bell burritos compete for shelf space and the school takes the profit. Still, the federal government now partially reimburses schools for the meals they provide, so it can skew that refund to subsidize healthier meals more generously. Nutritionists can also urge schools to forgo some of the profits on lower-fat foods in either the vending machine or the cafeteria and to charge more for high-fat foods to make up the difference. Kids will still gravitate to Papa John's, but they may at least add in an apple a day.

| *"The suggestion of adding a federal fat tax is ridiculous."*

Junk-Food Taxes Would Be Unfair and Ineffective

Pamela Parseghian

According to Pamela Parseghian in the following viewpoint, imposing taxes on high-calorie foods would be unfair and ineffective at reducing obesity in the United States. She maintains that, unlike cigarette smoke, which can harm non-smokers, indulging in unhealthy foods does not affect anyone other than the consumer. Therefore, she contends, the government has no right to regulate a person's food choices. Moreover, Parseghian argues that determining which foods have too much fat would be difficult, particularly in restaurants where recipes often vary. A veteran of the food industry, Parseghian has extensive professional experience in both restaurant operations and food writing.

As you read, consider the following questions:
1. According to the author, why was gluttony included in the seven deadly sins?
2. In the author's opinion, why is a fat tax a "class-specific tax"?
3. As reported by Parseghian, what is the National Restaurant Association's position on a fat tax?

Pamela Parseghian, "Support High-Calorie Food Tax Proposal? Fat Chance," *Nation's Restaurant News*, vol. 35, April 30, 2001, p. 44. Copyright © 2001 by Lebhar-Friedman, Inc. Reproduced by permission.

W ho needs [Jack] Kevorkian?[1] If what some nutritionists say about the deadly effect of our nation's high-
calorie diet is true, we should be able to take care of our own
mercy killing without the aid of a physician. Well-marbled
rib-eye steaks and a side of fries, untrimmed, veal breasts in
butter sauce, and roast ducks with sweetened toppings
should do the trick.

I admit that is a gruesome subject for a food column, but
I wanted to get your attention regarding a related matter. A
contingent of nutritionists has suggested that federal and all
local governments should impose a "small" tax on high-
calorie foods.

Michael Jacobson, Ph.D., of the Center for Science in the
Public Interest, Washington, D.C., and Kelly Brownell,
Ph.D., with the department of psychology, Yale University,
New Haven, Conn., wrote in the *American Journal of Public
Health*, "it has been suggested that foods high in calories, fat,
or sugar be subjected to special taxes and that the cost of
healthful foods, such as fruit and vegetables, be subsidized."

A Ridiculous Idea

Please. No matter how well funds are invested for improving society, the suggestion of adding a federal fat tax is
ridiculous. Our bodies, and what we put into them, are our
business as long as we don't hurt anyone else in the process.

It is easy to understand the control of alcohol consumption, since drunks can hurt innocent bystanders, especially
when they get behind the wheel. And taxing smokers makes
some sense, since secondhand smoke is a nuisance to those
of us who are not participating. But whom does a glutton
hurt? Does she take up too much space on the city bus or a
public sidewalk?

I admit that gluttony is one of the seven deadly sins, but
those rules were put down ages ago when food often was
scarce.

Personally, I was born at the wrong time. I can't go by a
painting of ladies with chubby cheeks and bulging bellies with-

---

1. Jack Kevorkian is a well-publicized physician who helped terminally ill patients
commit suicide.

out longing to have lived during an era when fat was the fad.

Now my friends look at their size 6 bodies and feel shame because their bellies aren't as flat as pancakes. One of those slim friends runs marathons and loves fast food. Should this lady be taxed for her weekly indulgence in french fries and a big burger? I don't think so. She probably could run circles around the nutrition Nazis suggesting such a tax.

An Unenforceable Proposal

Besides, how will anyone enforce the nonhealth-food taxes? Will it affect only the chain restaurants with preset recipes that are analyzed easily? How could anyone count calories in a fine-dining restaurant, where a line cook may throw an extra tablespoon of butter in a fish sauce one day? Who would know?

It is unfair if chain restaurants are attacked solely. What crime did they commit? Perhaps they did their jobs too well. They've mastered the art of offering flavorful and satisfying foods at an affordable price.

Lay Off the Twinkies

It's time to stand up for individual responsibility by insisting that Americans have the right to choose what we want to eat—and restaurants have the right to serve it. Our eating habits shouldn't be the government's business. Bureaucrats shouldn't be allowed to micromanage our menus or tax our Twinkies in the name of so-called public health.

David Bergland, *San Francisco Chronicle*, April 23, 2000.

Besides possibly hurting one segment of the industry more than any other, this is a class-specific tax. Mostly middle- and low-income folks patronize those affordable chain establishments, while the rich folks would continue to graze on foie gras, possibly without a levy.

The preposterous proposed tax sounds familiar to a former law. Remember the results of Prohibition?

How many illegal speakeasies were there? Now we'll have to churn butter in the bathtub and hide cows in our tool sheds.

I admit that I have a problem with folks with authority taking advantage of their power, so perhaps I'm overreacting a touch. Sure, subsidizing fresh fruits and vegetables is good. And the recent news of the Surgeon General's interest in combating obesity deserves applause. But how far will the lawmakers go? And will the public protest such a tax?

Oh yeah: A study conducted by the National Restaurant Association [NRA] found a whopping 92 percent of adults who were asked were opposed to high-calorie taxes. Steven Grover, vice president, Health and Safety Regulatory Affairs for the NRA, is dead set against the tax, as is the NRA as a whole. Grover says obesity is a complicated societal dilemma that simply cannot be controlled by such a simple tax.

So, like I said before, who needs Kevorkian?

I'd rather lessen the burden on my family and friends by taking the morbid matter into my own hands—send on a big bowl of fettuccine Alfredo with extra cheese, please.

> *"What we need is a national single-payer system that would eliminate unnecessary administrative costs, duplication and profits."*

Government-Funded Single-Payer Health Care Would Benefit America

Marcia Angell

According to Marcia Angell in the following viewpoint, the American health care system views health as a commodity. As a result, she argues, a large portion of the money paid for health care gets diverted from care to health care organizations' administrative and marketing costs and profits. A single-payer health care system, in which a new tax earmarked for health care would cover all health expenses for the nation, would eliminate unnecessary costs and ensure health coverage for everyone, Angell maintains. Angell, the former editor in chief of the *New England Journal of Medicine*, is a senior lecturer in social medicine at Harvard Medical School.

As you read, consider the following questions:
1. In the author's opinion, what is the criterion for receiving health care in the current system?
2. What dilemma have attempts to improve the system encountered, according to Angell?
3. How would an American single-payer system differ from the Canadian and British health care systems?

If it weren't for the steady beat of war drums [during the war in Iraq], health care would be front and center in [the] political debate. And war or no war, politicians will not be able to avoid it much longer. As John Breaux of Louisiana, long one of the most conservative Senate Democrats, recently told the press, "The system is collapsing around us."

Rising Costs

That is not hyperbole. Private health insurance premiums are rising at an unsustainable average of about 13 percent per year—and as much as 25 percent in some areas of the country. Coverage is shrinking, as more employers decide to cap their contributions to health insurance plans and workers find they cannot pay their rapidly expanding share. And with the rise in unemployment, more people are losing what limited coverage they had. [In September 2002], the Census Bureau reported that nearly 1.5 million Americans lost their insurance in 2001.

The fatal flaw in the system is that we treat health care as a commodity. That has been the case for a long time, but the effects were masked during the economic boom of the 1990's. Now, with the recession, the irrationality of that approach is exposed.

When health care becomes a commodity, the criterion for receiving it is ability to pay, not medical need. Private insurers and providers compete with one another to avoid getting stuck with high-cost patients, so they can keep more of their revenues. But this game of hot potato takes a lot of oversight and paperwork. In fact, the hallmark of the system is the extent to which health funds are diverted to overhead and profits.

Follow the Money

Look at what happens to the health-care dollar as it wends its way from employers to the doctors and hospitals that provide medical services. Private insurers regularly skim off the top 10 percent to 25 percent of premiums for administrative costs, marketing and profits. The remainder is passed along a gantlet of satellite businesses—insurance brokers, disease-management and utilization-review companies, lawyers, consultants, billing agencies, information management firms and so on. Their function is often to limit services in one way or another. They, too, take a cut, including enough for their own administrative costs, marketing and profits. As much as half the health-care dollar never reaches doctors and hospitals—who themselves face high overhead costs in dealing with multiple insurers.

One more absurdity of our market-based system: the pressure is to increase total health-care expenditures, not reduce them. Presumably, as a nation we want to constrain the growth of health costs. But that's simply not what health-care businesses do. Like all businesses, they want more, not fewer, customers—but only if they can pay.

Health Care Expenditures per Capita in 1997, Adjusted for Cost-of-Living Differences

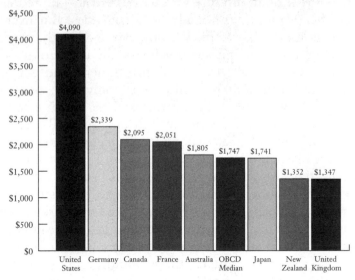

Gerard F. Anderson, "Multinational Comparisons of Health Care: Expenditures, Coverage, and Outcomes," The Commonwealth Fund, October 1998.

All piecemeal attempts to improve the system—while keeping it market-based—have run into the following dilemma: if access to services is expanded, costs rise; if costs are lowered, access is cut. That's the way it is. The only way to avoid this dilemma is to change the system entirely.

What we need is a national single-payer system that would eliminate unnecessary administrative costs, duplication and profits. In many ways, this would be tantamount to extending Medicare to the entire population. Medicare is, after all, a government-financed single-payer system embedded within our private, market-based system. It's by far the most efficient part of our health-care system, with overhead costs of less than 3 percent, and it covers virtually everyone over the age of 65. Medicare is not perfect, but it's the most popular part of the American health-care system.

Wasting Health Care Funds

Many people believe a single-payer system is a good idea, but that we can't afford it. The truth is that we can no longer afford not to have such a system. We now spend more than $5,000 a year on health care for each American—more than twice the average of other advanced countries. But nearly half that amount is wasted. We now pay for health care in multiple ways—through our paychecks, the prices of goods and services, taxes at all levels of government, and out-of-pocket fees. It makes more sense to pay only once, perhaps through a new tax on income earmarked for health care (in the same way Medicare is financed through payroll taxes).

It is sometimes argued that innovative technologies would be scarce in a national single-payer system, so we would have long waiting lists. This misconception is based on the fact that there are indeed waits for elective procedures in some countries with national health systems like Great Britain and Canada. But that's because they spend far less on health care than we do. If they were to put the same amount of money as we do into their systems, there would be no waits. For them, the problem is not the system; it's the money. For us, it's not the money; it's the system. We already spend enough for an excellent universal system.

A single-payer system is not socialized medicine. Although a new national program—like Medicare—would be publicly financed, the doctors and hospitals would not work for the government, but would remain private. Some fear onerous government regulations from a national payment system, but surely nothing could be more onerous for patients and providers than the multiple, intrusive regulations imposed on them by the private insurance industry today.

We live in a country that tolerates enormous disparities in income, material possessions and social privilege. That may be inevitable in a free-market economy. But those disparities should not extend to essential services like education, clean water and air and protection from crime, all of which we already acknowledge are public responsibilities. The same should be true for medical care—particularly since we can well afford to provide it for everyone if we end the waste and profiteering of our market-based system.

"*A single-payer system has not worked well anywhere in the world.*"

Government-Funded Single-Payer Health Care Would Not Benefit America

David C. MacDonald

In the following viewpoint David C. MacDonald argues that a single-payer health system, in which universal health care is subsidized by a federal tax, would severely limit an individual's options regarding care. He contends that patients, not the government, should control where their health care dollars are spent. Returning control to the patient, MacDonald maintains, would help keep health care costs down and ensure quality care. MacDonald is a practicing physician and a founder of the American Association of Patients and Providers, a nonprofit membership organization.

As you read, consider the following questions:

1. How is a single-payer system similar to a managed care system, in the author's opinion?
2. Why are medical policies comparable to car insurance policies, as stated by MacDonald?
3. As reported by the author, what are the benefits of the Cares for America program?

Imagine this scenario: You just purchased a new car. The salesperson explains that all new-car owners must participate in a new program: "Managed Car." This is an attempt to cut down on the paperwork and waste associated with the operation of an automobile. Your service representative will help you locate the "best" (cheapest) oil to buy and the "best" (cheapest) service locations participating in their program and will help you avoid costly, preventive maintenance. They also will help you avoid those who might take advantage of you by recommending wasteful additives or synthetic oils that are more expensive and outside the mainstream of auto maintenance.

Sound ridiculous? I agree, but the above is a close parallel to what would happen under a single-payer health-insurance program. Imagine another scenario: You walk into the grocery store and there is a sign at the entrance stating that there is a new program for the county, the "County Single-Payer Food Program," for all county residents. After all, food is a right and our country should not let anyone starve to death. Food prices no longer would be posted, for fear that the store managers might compromise their commitment to their customers. So you meander through the store and you enjoy purchasing without regard for the cost of the products. In fact, it is not long before your food selections change from previous trips to the same store. The T-bone steaks seem more attractive, the lobster finds its way into your basket and you pass by the day-old bread section you used to frequent. As you enter the checkout line the cashier presents you with the total bill: $110.89. You present your Single-Payer Food Group card, the cashier makes a note on the receipt and you leave the store. Six months later, the Single-Payer County Food Group writes to you stating they mailed a check to the grocery store for $37.65, the usual and customary amount for the food you purchased.

Facing Reality

These scenarios are not far from the reality of what managed-care organizations have done to our health-care system and how a single-payer system may function. Our society never would let the government determine where our car should be serviced, the type of gasoline we may buy and how often we are able to change the oil in our car. Why do we let this happen with our health care?

What is so attractive about a single-payer system? For the patients, there is the perception that whenever they are ill, a medical facility will be waiting with open arms to take care of them. For the physicians, there is the lure of less paperwork and the freedom to practice their art without the complexities associated with billing. For the politicians, healthcare decisions attract voters who are hopeful that somehow the central government will be able to stabilize the fear of our ailing health-care system. Many who are not familiar with the actual health-care delivery system in other countries often cite partial truths that imply the grass is greener in a single-payer environment. Many use Canada as a country for the United States to emulate, without knowing how their system functions. [On] January 2, [2000,] 23 of the 25 hospital emergency rooms in Toronto were closed to patients, regardless of the severity of their illness. Canada has long waiting lists for medical technology such as MRI and CT scanners. According to the Vancouver-based Fraser Institute, studies show that in 1997–98 about 170,000 people in British Columbia were not covered because they had not paid premiums required by the province. Alberta also requires a premium and does not cover individuals who do not pay. A 1999 poll found that 76 percent of Canadians now believe the health-care system is in crisis.

Those who favor a central-government single-payer system often cite the millions who are uninsured as the main reason for the need for universal coverage. However, the number of uninsured is a very soft number. According to the U.S. Census Bureau, in 1998 3.5 million of the uninsured had incomes that exceeded $75,000/year. According to a 1996 survey, 6.3 million had access to health insurance and chose not to pay for it. Actually, medical costs are low for most of us, according to the *Journal of American Health Policy*. They report that 33 percent of the U.S. population have no medical expenses each year. Another 40 percent spend less than $500 per year and only 3 percent spend more than $5,000 per year. A question we must consider is: Are we paying inflated fees for insurance that is not paying for what Americans are asking for?

Theoretical Arguments

The stark reality is a single-payer system has not worked well anywhere in the world. Why do some Americans believe we can make it work here? As a practicing family physician, it is frustrating to listen to theoretical arguments for a single-payer system. A far different reality belies the theory, such as the university hospital in the Southwest that advertised for much of the local surgical business. Not long after a successful advertising campaign, they realized that they could not perform the procedures for the price they advertised.

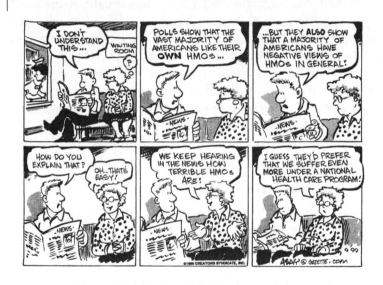

Asay. © 1999 by Creators Syndicate, Inc. Reprinted with permission.

Ironically, managed-care systems function much like a single-payer program because decisions are made at a distance from the consumer. A study by Deloitte and Touche, a consulting firm, found that consumers are not satisfied with managed care. Sixty-two percent believe HMOs [Health Maintenance Organizations] make it harder to see specialists; 61 percent believe they have less time with their patients in an HMO environment; and 43 percent are not satisfied with access to their physician. According to the *Yankelovich Monitor*, 70 percent of physicians surveyed characterized themselves as against managed care; 46 percent often think about leaving clinical practice; and the hassle factor has increased due to restrictions on the ability to treat, cumbersome preauthorization and prolonged reimbursement time. California certainly has had challenges with health care. According to Price Waterhouse, health-care premiums continue to increase despite declining payments to the physicians. Patients, physicians and politicians are so frustrated that many are ready to accept anything that may provide relief.

Most patients and providers are unaware of the actual costs for clinic visits, hospitalizations, procedures and medications. As a result, the utilization rate for services usually is distorted. Some services may be underutilized, such as preventive care, or others may be overutilized, such as emergency rooms. Studies have found that if the patient participation is high enough (with additional charges for after-hour services), the utilization rate declines. Some of the positive aspects that have surfaced as a result of managed care are the waste and inflated fees for some services. Physicians, hospitals, vendors, research projects, patients and pharmaceutical companies are all responsible for our inflated health-care costs.

The Insurance Umbrella

Major medical policies are [similarly affordable] to high-deductible car insurance. If we had insurance to cover our gasoline, tires and wiper blades, our car insurance would be outrageous. In essence, health insurance is so expensive because we are trying to insure services and products that should not fall under the insurance umbrella. Small-business owners constantly are trying to find a reasonable health-insurance program for their employees. As a result, some employees change health plans yearly. Continuity of care is lost, patient choice is almost unheard of and premiums continue to increase while satisfaction wanes.

Another reality is that costs have increased in all aspects of society. A recent visit by my plumber reminded me that outpatient health-care costs are no more expensive than other services provided. The fear of the major medical events is what drives us all to purchase health insurance.

However, there is a single-payer system that requires no legislation to implement, already has demonstrated its ability to control costs, empowers patient choice, maintains individual privacy and increases access to care. Who is the single payer in this system? The patient! Patients are the best ones to determine the type of health care they should receive. If patients have the incentive to remain well, and if they have access to unspent health-care dollars, they will make very wise health-care decisions.

Patients' Choice

My partner, Dr. Vern Cherewatenko, and I started a non-profit group, the American Association of Patients and Providers, to develop solutions to our health-care dilemma that are not a burden to the taxpayers. One program, SimpleCare, eliminates the administrative waste and passes the savings back to the patient. This program initially was developed to help the uninsured. However, the program is also a boon to consumers who have a major medical policy and would like to retain the decision-making authority regarding their health-care dollars. Patients are able to decide the integrative-medicine aspects that meet their needs without the hassle of preauthorization. Patients and providers are thrilled with this program.

Another nonprofit program developed for the uninsured or those who are unable to pay is Cares for America. Patients are seen and a charge generated similar to SimpleCare. The patient then has 90 days to volunteer his or her time with participating community programs. Takin' It to the Streets is a similar program. Providers bring health care to a needy part of the community in exchange for work, such as sweeping the streets, picking up trash or planting flowers.

As employers continue to get out of the health-care industry, there are fewer options for individuals. We should allow the free market to establish the "true" insurance costs by removing the mandated benefits. We also should remove the barrier for medical-savings accounts and allow patients to determine where their health-care dollars are spent.

Periodical Bibliography

The following articles have been selected to supplement the diverse views presented in this chapter.

Sue Blevins
"Individuals Lose but Government and Corporations Gain Control over Personal Health and Genetic Information," *Institute for Health Freedom*, August 12, 2002.

Fred H. Cate
"Principles for Protecting Privacy," *Cato Journal*, Spring/Summer 2002.

Tom A. Coburn
"Patients' Rights, Done Wrong," *New York Times*, July 30, 1999.

Consumer Freedom
"Fat Tax Attack! Nannies Renew Push for a Twinkie Tax," August 1, 2000.

Larry Elder
"Coming Soon: The Fat Tax," *Capitalism Magazine*, November 9, 1999.

Suzanne Gordon
"Perspective on Managed Care: The Doctor Can't See You Now: HMOs Defeat Their Claim to Preventive Medicine with Huge Patient Loads on Clinicians," *Los Angeles Times*, July 6, 1999.

Thomas W. Hazlett
"HMO Phobia: Quack Remedies for the Health Care 'Crisis,'" *Reason*, February 1999.

Gerald F. Kreyche
"Are We Obsessed About Our Health?" *USA Today*, July 2000.

Kate O'Beirne
"Poor and Fat," *National Review*, February 10, 2003.

Kathleen O'Connor
"Desperately in Search of a Health Care Blueprint," *Seattle Times*, November 23, 2001.

Adam Oliver, Andrew Healey, and Julian Le Grand
"Addressing Health Care Inequalities," *Lancet*, August 17, 2002.

Jonathan Rauch
"The Fat Tax: A Modest Proposal," *Atlantic Monthly*, December 2002.

Kevin W. Wildes
"Patient No More: Why Did the Golden Age of Medicine Collapse?" *America*, July 16, 2001.

For Further Discussion

Chapter 1

1. The American Cancer Society (ACS) argues that smoking causes heart disease, cancer, emphysema, and numerous other maladies. Eric Boyd maintains that antismoking activists have exaggerated the health risks of smoking. Whose argument do you find most convincing and why?

2. According to Tom Farley and Deborah Cohen, recommendations by health experts to eat less and exercise more have failed to reduce the problem of obesity in America. To combat the epidemic of obesity, Farley and Cohen suggest reducing the availability of junk food, increasing access to healthy fruits and vegetables, and encouraging people to walk or cycle instead of drive. Do you think these measures would be successful? Citing from the text, explain your answer.

3. Glenn Gaesser contends that problems commonly associated with obesity, such as heart disease, high blood pressure, and diabetes, are caused by lifestyle choices, not a person's weight. He argues that a sedentary thin person who eats a lot of high fat foods is less healthy than a heavy person who exercises and eats healthfully. Do you agree with his argument? Cite from his viewpoint while constructing your answer.

4. Jonny Bowden asserts that the American diet does not provide sufficient vitamins and minerals. Vitamin supplements, he argues, are essential for good health, Colin Brennan maintains that a healthy diet supplies most people with the vitamins and minerals necessary for good health; thus he argues that vitamin supplements are unnecessary. With whose argument do you most agree? Explain your answer.

Chapter 2

1. According to JoAnn Manson, exercise is associated with a lower risk of disease and improves mental functioning. Rebecca Prussin, Philip Harvey, and Theresa Foy DiGeronimo warn that exercising can be addicting and lead to injuries and emotional problems. In your own experience, has exercise been a benefit or detriment to your quality of life? Citing from the text and your experience, explain why or why not.

2. According to James Guest and Marvin M. Lipman, the weight-loss herb ephedra poses serious health risks, such as heart attacks and strokes. In Barbara Zeitlin Kravets's opinion, ephedra is the most effective weight-loss aid available, and contends that its

risks have been exaggerated. With whose argument do you most agree? Explain.

Chapter 3

1. Susan Ince argues that some alternative therapies, such as acupuncture and hypnosis, have proven health benefits. Roland J. Lamarine maintains that alternative therapies are not submitted to the rigorous testing that conventional remedies are and therefore can be dangerous. With whose argument do you most agree? Explain your answer.

2. According to Eric L. Foxman, homeopathy enhances the body's healing system without the unpleasant side effects of conventional drugs. Stephen Barrett argues that the amount of medicine in homeopathic treatments is too small to have any effect on the patient, and any relief the patient feels is due to the placebo effect. Examine the evidence offered by both authors and construct your own opinion about whether or not homeopathy has healing powers.

3. In Anne McIntyre's opinion, herbal supplements relieve a number of physical and mental ailments and slow down the aging process. John M. Allen contends that herbal supplements can be dangerous because they are not subjected to the same testing and labeling as pharmaceutical drugs. Whose evidence do you find most convincing and why?

4. Gregg Easterbrook maintains that religious faith is associated with fewer health problems and a longer lifespan. Richard P. Sloan, Emilia Bagiella, and Tia Powell argue that a link between religious faith and better health has not been proven. In your experience, are religious people more healthy? Citing from the text and your own experience, explain why or why not.

Chapter 4

1. Hanna Rosin argues that higher taxes on fat- and sugar-laden foods would encourage people to purchase healthier foods such as fruits and vegetables. Pamela Parseghian contends the government has no right to regulate a person's food choices. Considering the authors' opinions, formulate your own argument about whether junk-food taxes would be effective.

2. According to Marcia Angell, government-funded single-payer health care would reduce health care costs and eliminate the problem of uninsured Americans. David C. MacDonald maintains that single-payer health care would reduce patient control over health care options. Whose argument do you find most convincing? Explain.

Organizations to Contact

The editors have compiled the following list of organizations concerned with the issues debated in this book. The descriptions are derived from materials provided by the organizations. All have publications or information available for interested readers. The list was compiled on the date of publication of the present volume; names, addresses, and phone numbers may change. Be aware that many organizations take several weeks or longer to respond to inquiries, so allow as much time as possible.

American Association of Retired People (AARP)
601 E Street NW, Washington, DC 20049
(800) 424-3410
website: www.aarp.org

AARP is a nonprofit, nonpartisan membership organization for people fifty years of age and over. They provide information and resources; advocate on legislative, consumer, and legal issues; assist members to serve their communities; and offer a wide range of unique benefits, special products, and services for members. These benefits include AARP Webplace at www.aarp.org, *AARP Modern Maturity* and *My Generation* magazines, the monthly *AARP Bulletin*, and a Spanish-language newspaper, *Segunda Juventud*. Active in every state, the District of Columbia, Puerto Rico, and the U.S. Virgin Islands, AARP celebrates the attitude that age is just a number and life is what you make it.

American Chiropractic Association (ACA)
1701 Clarendon Blvd., Arlington, VA 22209
(800) 986-4636 • fax: (703) 243-2593
e-mail: memberinfo@amerchiro.org • website: www.amerchiro.org

ACA promotes legislation defining chiropractic health care and works to increase the public's awareness and use of chiropractic medicine. Its publications include the monthly *Journal of the American Chiropractic Association* and the monthly newsletter *ACA Today*.

American College of Sports Medicine (ACSM)
PO Box 1440, Indianapolis, IN 46202
(317) 637-9200 • fax: (317) 634-7817
e-mail: vbragg@acsm.org • website: www.acsm.org

ACSM conducts research on sports medicine and exercise science to discover how they can enhance physical performance, fitness, and health. It publishes the quarterly newsletter *Sports Medicine Bulletin*, the monthly journal *Medicine and Science in Sports and Ex-*

ercise, the *ACSM Health and Fitness Journal*, and various monographs in its annual *Exercise and Sport Sciences Review.*

American Council on Science and Health (ACSH)
1995 Broadway, 2nd Fl., New York, NY 10023-5860
(212) 362-7044 • fax: (212) 362-4919
e-mail: whelan@acsh.org • website: www.acsh.org
ACSH provides consumers with scientifically balanced evaluations of food, chemicals, the environment, and human health. It publishes the quarterly magazine *Priorities for Health*, the semiannual *News from ACSH*, the book *Issues in Nutrition*, and the booklets *Aspirin and Health* and *Does Moderate Alcohol Consumption Prolong Life?*

American Dietetic Association (ADA)
120 S. Riverside Plaza, Suite 2000, Chicago, IL 60606
(312) 899-0040 • fax: (312) 899-1979
e-mail: adaf@eatright.org • website: www.eatright.org
ADA is the largest organization of food and nutrition professionals in the United States. It works to shape the food choices and nutritional status of the public for optimal nutrition, health, and well-being. The association publishes the monthly *Journal of the American Dietetic Association* as well as a variety of booklets, pamphlets, and fact sheets about nutrition.

American Holistic Medical Association (AHMA)
12101 Menaul Blvd. NE, Suite C, Albuquerque, NM 87112
(505) 292-7788 • fax: (505) 293-7582
e-mail: info@holisticmedicine.org
website: www.holisticmedicine.org
AHMA promotes the practice of holistic health care, a concept that emphasizes the integration of physical, mental, emotional, and spiritual concerns with environmental harmony. AHMA publishes a quarterly newsletter.

American Medical Association (AMA)
515 N. State St., Chicago, IL 60610
(312) 464-5000
website: www.ama-assn.org
The AMA is the primary professional association of physicians in the United States. Founded in 1847, it disseminates information to its members and the public concerning medical breakthroughs, medical and health legislation, educational standards for physicians, and other issues concerning medicine and health care. The AMA operates a library and offers many publications, including

the weekly *JAMA: The Journal of the American Medical Association*, the weekly newspaper *American Medical News*, and journals covering specific medical specialties.

American Public Health Association (APHA)
800 I St. NW, Washington, DC 20001
(302) 777-2742 • fax: (202) 777-2534
e-mail: comments@apha.org • website: www.apha.org

APHA works to protect and promote personal, mental, and environmental health by establishing health standards and researching public health issues. In addition to books, manuals, and pamphlets, the association's publications service offers the monthly *American Journal of Public Health* and the *Nation's Health*, which is published ten times per year.

American Society of Law, Medicine, and Ethics (ASLME)
765 Commonwealth Ave., Suite 1634, Boston, MA 02215
(617) 262-4990 • fax: (617) 437-7596
e-mail: info@aslme.org • website: www.aslme.org

ASLME members include physicians, attorneys, health care administrators, and others interested in the relationship between law and medicine and in health law. The organization has an information clearinghouse and a library. It publishes the quarterlies *American Journal of Law and Medicine* and the *Journal of Law, Medicine, and Ethics*.

Brookings Institution
1775 Massachusetts Ave. NW, Washington, DC 20036-2188
(202) 797-6105 • fax: (202) 797-2495
e-mail: brookinfo@brookings.edu • website: www.brook.edu

Founded in 1927, the institution is a liberal research and education organization that publishes material on economics, government, and foreign policy. It strives to serve as a bridge between scholarship and public policy, bringing new knowledge to the attention of decision makers and providing scholars with improved insight into public policy issues. The Brookings Institution produces hundreds of abstracts and reports on health care, with topics ranging from Medicaid to persons with disabilities.

Cato Institute
1000 Massachusetts Ave. NW, Washington, DC 20001-5403
(202) 842-0200 • fax: (202) 842-3490
e-mail: cato@cato.org • website: www.cato.org

The institute is a libertarian public policy research foundation dedicated to limiting the role of government and protecting individual liberties. Its Health and Welfare Studies department works to formulate and popularize a free-market agenda for health care reform. The institute publishes the quarterly magazine *Regulation*, the bimonthly *Cato Policy Report*, and numerous books and commentaries, hundreds of which relate to health care.

Center for Studying Health System Change (HSC)
600 Maryland Ave. SW, #550, Washington, DC
(202) 484-5261 • fax: (202) 484-9258
e-mail: hscinfo@hschange.org • website: www.hschange.org

The Center for Studying Health System Change (HSC) is a nonpartisan policy research organization located in Washington, D.C. HSC designs and conducts studies focused on the U.S health care system to inform the thinking and decisions of policy makers in government and private industry. In addition to this applied use, HSC studies contribute more broadly to the body of health care policy research that enables decision makers to understand change and the national and local market forces driving that change. They publish issue briefs, community reports, tracking reports, data bulletins, and journal articles based on their research.

Consumers Union
101 Truman Ave., Yonkers, NY 10703-1057
(914) 378-2000 • fax: (914) 378-2455
website: www.consumersunion.org

Consumers Union, publisher of *Consumer Reports*, is an independent, nonprofit testing and information organization serving only consumers. They are a comprehensive source for unbiased advice about products and services, personal finance, health, health care, nutrition, and other consumer concerns. Since 1936, they have been testing products, informing the public, and protecting consumers.

Healthcare Leadership Council (HLC)
900 17th Street NW, Suite 600, Washington, DC 20006
(202) 452-8700 • fax: (202) 296-9561
e-mail: mgrealy@hlc.org • website: www.hlc.org

The council is a forum in which health care industry leaders can jointly develop policies, plans, and programs that support a market-based health care system. HLC believes America's health care system should value innovation and provide affordable high-quality health care free from excessive government regulations. It offers the latest press releases on health issues and several public policy papers with titles such as "Empowering Consumers and Patients" and "Ensuring Responsible Government."

The Heritage Foundation
214 Massachusetts Ave. NE, Washington, DC 20002
(202) 546-4400 • fax: (202) 546-8328
e-mail: info@heritage.org • website: www.heritage.org

The Heritage Foundation is a public policy research institute that supports limited government and the free market system. It opposes nationalized health care and has proposed its own health care reform plan that minimizes government involvement. The foundation publishes the quarterly journal *Policy Review* as well as monographs, books, and papers concerning health care in America.

Institute for Health Freedom (IHF)
1825 Eye St. NW, Washington, DC 20036
(202) 429-6610 • fax: (202) 861-1973
e-mail: feedback@forhealthfreedom.org
website: www.forhealthfreedom.org

The institute is a nonpartisan, nonprofit research center established to bring the issues of personal freedom in choosing health care to the forefront of America's health policy debate. Its mission is to present the ethical and economic case for strengthening personal health freedom. IHF's research and analyses are published as policy briefings on subjects such as "Children's Health Care," "Monopoly in Medicine," and "Legal Issues." All are available through its website.

Kaiser Family Foundation
2400 Sand Hill Rd., Menlo Park, CA 94025
(650) 854-9400 • fax: (650) 854-4800
website: www.kff.org

The Henry J. Kaiser Family Foundation is an independent philanthropy focusing on the major health care issues facing the nation. The foundation is an independent voice and source of facts and analysis for policy makers, the media, the health care community, and the general public. It is primarily an operating organization that develops and runs its own research and communications programs, often in partnership with outside organizations. The foundation contracts with a wide range of outside individuals and organizations through its programs and also continues to make a small number of grants for unsolicited proposals each year. Foundation work is focused in three main areas: Health Policy, Media and Public Education, and Health and Development in South

Africa. The foundation publishes hundreds of papers, articles, and reports each year. Most are available through its website.

National Association to Advance Fat Acceptance (NAAFA)
PO Box 188620, Sacramento, CA 95818
(916) 558-6880 • fax: (916) 558-6881
e-mail: mbnaafa@aol.com • website: www.naafa.org
NAAFA works through public education and activism to end weight-based discrimination and to improve the quality of life for overweight people. The association provides information about the disadvantages of weight-loss treatments and publishes the bimonthly *NAAFA Newsletter.*

National Cattlemen's Beef Association (NCBA)
9110 E. Nichols Ave., Suite 300, Centennial, CO 80112
(303) 694-0305 • fax: (303) 694-2851
e-mail: cattle@beef.org • website: www.beef.org
NCBA is a service organization for livestock marketers, growers, meat packers, food retailers, and food service firms. It works to promote and educate the public about the meat industry, beef nutrition, and food safety. NCBA publishes the *Food and Nutrition News* five times per year, as well as numerous brochures and pamphlets.

National Center for Complementary and Alternative Medicine (NCCAM)
NCCAM Clearinghouse, PO Box 7923, Gaithersburg, MD 20898
(888) 644-6226 • fax: (866) 464-3616
e-mail: info@nccam.nih.gov • website: nccam.nih.gov
NCCAM is one of twenty-seven institutes that make up the National Institutes of Health (NIH). Their mission is to support research on complementary and alternative medicine (CAM), and to disseminate information to the public and professionals on which CAM modalities work, which do not, and why. NCCAM publishes a quarterly newsletter, *Complementary and Alternative Medicine at the NIH.*

National Coalition on Health Care
1200 G Street NW, Suite 750, Washington, DC 20005
(202) 638-7151 • fax: (202) 638-7166
e-mail: info@nchc.org • website: www.nchc.org
The National Coalition on Health Care is a nonprofit, nonpartisan group that represents the nation's largest alliance working to improve America's health care and make it more affordable. The coalition offers several policy studies with titles ranging from "Why

the Quality of U.S. Health Care Must Be Improved" to "The Rising Number of Uninsured Workers: An Approaching Crisis in Health Care Financing."

National Strength and Conditioning Association (NSCA)
PO Box 9908, Colorado Springs, CO 80932
(719) 632-6722 • fax: (719) 632-6367
e-mail: nsca@nsca-lift.org • website: www.nsca-lift.org

NSCA encourages the use of strength and conditioning techniques for improved physical performance. It publishes the bimonthly journal *Strength and Conditioning*, the quarterly *Journal of Strength and Conditioning Research*, and the bimonthly newsletter *NSCA Bulletin*.

North American Vegetarian Society (NAVS)
PO Box 72, Dolgeville, NY 13329
(518) 568-7970 • fax: (518) 568-7636
e-mail: navs@telenet.net • website: www.navs-online.org

NAVS works to educate the public and the media about the nutritional, economical, ecological, and ethical benefits of a vegetarian diet. Its publications include the quarterly magazine *Vegetarian Voice* and the books *Good Nutrition: A Look at Vegetarian Basics*, *Vegetarianism: Answers to the Most Commonly Asked Questions*, and *Vegetarianism: Tipping the Scales for the Environment*.

Urban Institute
2100 M St. NW, Washington, DC 20037
(202) 261-5244
e-mail: paffairs@ui.urban.org • website: www.urban.org

The Urban Institute investigates social and economic problems confronting the nation and analyzes efforts to solve these problems. In addition, it works to improve government decisions and their implementations and to increase citizen awareness about important public choices. It offers a wide variety of resources, including books such as *Restructuring Medicare: Impacts on Beneficiaries* and *The Decline in Medical Spending Growth in 1996: Why Did It Happen?*

U.S. Food and Drug Administration (FDA)
5600 Fishers Ln., Rockville, MD 20857
toll free: (888) 463-6332
website: www.fda.gov

The FDA is a consumer protection agency that is responsible for inspecting foods and drugs to ensure their quality and safety.

Through its Center for Food Safety and Applied Nutrition, the FDA researches and develops standards for the quality, nutrition, and safety of foods and drugs. Publications available from the FDA and the Center for Food Safety and Applied Nutrition include the magazine *FDA Consumer* and the information packets *FDA: Safeguarding America's Health, Facts About Weight Loss: Products and Programs, Nutrition and the Elderly*, and *Vegetarian Diets: The Pluses and the Pitfalls.*

Bibliography of Books

Sandra Alters   *Essential Concepts for Healthy Living*. Boston: Jones & Bartlett, 2003.

Norman B. Anderson and P. Elizabeth Anderson   *Emotional Longevity: What Really Determines How Long You Live*. New York: Viking, 2003.

F. Batmanghelidj   *Water: For Your Health, for Healing, for Life: You're Not Sick, You're Thirsty!* New York: Warner, 2003.

Marty Becker   *The Healing Power of Pets: Harnessing the Amazing Ability of Pets to Make and Keep People Healthy*. New York: Hyperion, 2003.

Mark Blumenthal   *The ABC Clinical Guide to Herbs*. New York: Thieme Medical Publishers, 2003.

Cheryl Canfield   *Profound Healing: The Power of Acceptance on the Path to Wellness*. Rochester, VT: Inner Traditions, 2003.

James R. Carey   *Longevity: The Biology and Demography of Life Span*. Princeton, NJ: Princeton University Press, 2003.

Jane Cicchetti   *Dreams, Symbols, and Homeopathy: Archetypal Dimensions of Healing*. Berkeley, CA: North Atlantic, 2003.

Larry P. Credit   *Your Guide to Alternative Medicine*. Garden City, NY: Square One, 2003.

Greg Crister   *Fat Land: How Americans Became the Fattest People in the World*. Boston: Houghton Mifflin, 2003.

Catherine Cumming   *The Little Book of Color Healing: Energy*. London: Mitchell Beazley, 2002.

Larry Dossey   *Healing Beyond the Body Medicine and the Infinite Reach of the Mind*. Boston: Shambhala, 2003.

Carl Elliott   *Better than Well: American Medicine Meets the American Dream*. New York: W.W. Norton, 2003.

Steven R. Feikin and Liz Zozanello Emery   *The Complete Book of Diet Drugs: Everything You Need to Know About Today's Prescription and Over-the-Counter Weight Loss Products*. New York: Kensington, 2000.

Glenn A. Gaesser and Steven N. Blair   *Big Fat Lies: The Truth About Your Weight and Health*. Carlsbad, CA: Gurze, 2002.

Thomas E. Getzen   *Health Economics: Fundamentals and Flow of Funds.* Hoboken, NJ: John Wiley, 2003.

Colin Gordon   *Dead on Arrival: The Politics of Healthcare in Twentieth-Century America.* Princeton, NJ: Princeton University Press, 2003.

Bob Greene   *Get with the Program! Guide to Good Eating: Great Food for Health.* New York: Simon and Schuster, 2003.

Deborah Haas-Wilson   *Managed Care and Monopoly Power: The Antitrust Challenge.* Boston: Harvard University Press, 2003.

Letha Hadady   *Healthy Beauty: Using Nature's Secrets to Look Great and Feel Terrific.* Hoboken, NJ: John Wiley, 2003.

David U. Himmelstein   *Bleeding the Patient Dry.* Monroe, ME: Common Courage, 2003.

Frank W. Hoffman   *Herbal Medicine and Botanical Medical Fads.* Binghampton, NY: Haworth, 2003.

Edward J. Jackowski   *Escape Your Shape: How to Work Out Smarter, Not Harder.* New York: Simon and Schuster, 2001.

Roger Jahnke   *The Healing Promise of Qi: Creating Extraordinary Wellness with Qigong and Tai-Chi.* New York: McGraw-Hill, 2002.

R. Klettke   *A Guy's Gotta Eat: The Regular Guy's Guide to Eating Smart.* New York: Marlowe, 2003.

Claire Kowalchik   *The Complete Book of Running for Women: Everything You Need to Know About Training, Nutrition, Injury Prevention, Motivation, Racing, and Much, Much More.* New York: Simon and Schuster, 1999.

Walt L. Larimore   *10 Essentials of Highly Healthy People.* Grand Rapids, MI: Zondervan, 2002.

Michael Lenarz   *Chiropractic Way: How Chiropractic Care Can Stop Your Pain and Help You Regain Your Health Without Drugs or Surgery.* New York: Bantam, 2003.

Elinor Levy   *New Killer Diseases: How the Alarming Evolution of Mutant Germs Threatens Us All.* New York: Crown, 2003.

Shari Lieberman   *The Real Vitamin and Mineral Book.* New York: Penguin Putnam, 2003.

Jan McCray   *Your Redemptive Healing: Experience God's Freedom, Wholeness, and Blessing.* Grand Rapids, MI: Chosen, 2003.

Earl L. Mindell   *Prescription Alternatives: Hundreds of Safe, Natural Prescription-Free Remedies to Restore and Maintain Your Health.* Columbus, OH: McGraw-Hill, 2003.

Caroline Myss   *Anatomy of the Spirit: The Seven Stages of Power and Healing.* New York: Random House, 1997.

Marion Nestle   *Food Politics: How the Food Industry Influences Nutrition and Health.* Berkeley: University of California Press, 2002.

David M. Nganele   *The Best Healthcare for Less: Saving Money on Chronic Medical Care and Prescription Drugs.* Hoboken, NJ: John Wiley, 2003.

Carol Emery Normadi and Laurelee Roark   *It's Not About Food: Change Your Mind, Change Your Life, End Your Obsession with Food and Weight.* New York: Berkley, 1999.

Bill Pearl   *Getting Stronger: Weight Training for Men and Women.* Bolinas, CA: Shelter, 2001.

Lorraine Perretta   *Brain Food: The Essential Guide to Boosting Brain Power.* London: Hamlyn, 2002.

Bill Phillips   *Body for Life: 12 Weeks to Mental and Physical Strength.* New York: HarperCollins, 1999.

Michael S. Richardson   *Health Basics: A Doctor's Plainspoken Advice About How Your Body Works and What to Do When It Doesn't.* Chester, NJ: Next Decade, 2003.

Eric Schlosser   *Fast Food Nation: The Dark Side of the All-American Meal.* New York: HarperCollins, 2002.

Christina Sell and Karuna Fedorschak   *Yoga from the Inside Out: Making Peace with Your Body Through Yoga.* Prescott, AZ: Hohm, 2003.

Jay W. Shelton   *Homeopathy: How It Really Works.* Amherst, NY: Prometheus, 2003.

Thomas J. Slaga   *The Detox Revolution.* New York: McGraw-Hill, 2003.

Frank A. Sloan   *The Smoking Puzzle: Information, Risk Perception, and Choice.* Boston: Harvard University Press, 2003.

Barbara J. Sowada   *Call to Be Whole: The Fundamentals of Healthcare Reform.* Westport, CT: Greenwood, 2003.

Sandra Steingraber   *Having Faith.* New York: Berkley, 2003.

Shawn M. Talbott   *Guide to Understanding Dietary Supplements: Magic Bullets or Modern Snake Oil?* Binghampton, NY: Haworth, 2002.

Pamela Walker   *Understanding the Risks of Diet Drugs.* New York:
                        Rosen, 2000.

Roanne Weisman   *Own Your Health: Choosing the Best from Alterna-
                        tive and Conventional Medicine.* Deerfield Beach,
                        FL: Health Communications, 2003.

Arthur H. White   *The Posture Prescription: A Doctor's RX for Elimi-
                        nating Back, Muscle, and Joint Pain, Achieving
                        Optimum Strength and Mobility, Living a Lifetime
                        of Fitness and Wellbeing.* New York: Crown,
                        2003.

Index